My Mother's Roommate

My Mother's Roommate

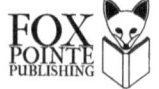

A posthumous memoir by Sandra Ann Cowden
with a forward and epilogue by Dr. Karen Cowden Dahl

Copyright © 2024 by Karen Cowden Dahl

All rights reserved. Published in the United States by Fox Pointe Publishing, LLP. No part of this book may be reproduced in any form or by any electronic or mechanical means, including information storage and retrieval systems, without permission in writing from the publisher.

This book is a memoir. It contains the author's mother's memories of her personal experiences from her perspective. Some names have been changed and some dialogue has been recreated. This book also discusses medical themes, but no part of the book is intended as medical advice. The reader should consult with their doctor in any matters relating to their health.

www.foxpointepublishing.com/author-karen-cowden-dahl

Library of Congress Cataloging-in-Publication Data

Cowden Dahl, Karen, author.
Olson, Sarah, editor.
Wagner, Kylie, designer.

My Mother's Roommate / Karen Cowden Dahl. – First edition.

Summary: The memoir of a woman with cancer, prefaced and followed by the memories and medical understanding of her daughter, a cancer researcher.

ISBN 978-1-955743-93-8 (hardcover) / 979-8-9938504-8-1 (softcover)

[1. Personal Memoirs – Biography & Autobiography. 2. Medical – Biography & Autobiography. 3. Motherhood – Family & Relationships.]

Library of Congress Control Number: 2 0 2 3 9 5 1 6 0 2

Second Printing April 2026

If my mom, Sandra, had finished her autobiography, she would have dedicated her story to her husband, Bob Cowden. He was her strength during her darkest hours. Thank you, Daddy! Thank you for loving my mom and taking care of my mom, my brother, and me. All my love~

To the cancer patients who are fighting: You are our purpose. After her cancer diagnosis, Sandra dedicated herself to helping other cancer patients with their pain and trauma. Sandra started this book to connect with patients as she pursued her master's degree in counseling to serve patients. My life's work is to conduct cancer research. I dream that my research leads to answers and healing and my mother's memoir offers comfort and hope.

To the cancer angels: You are THE inspiration. We miss you. You are never forgotten.

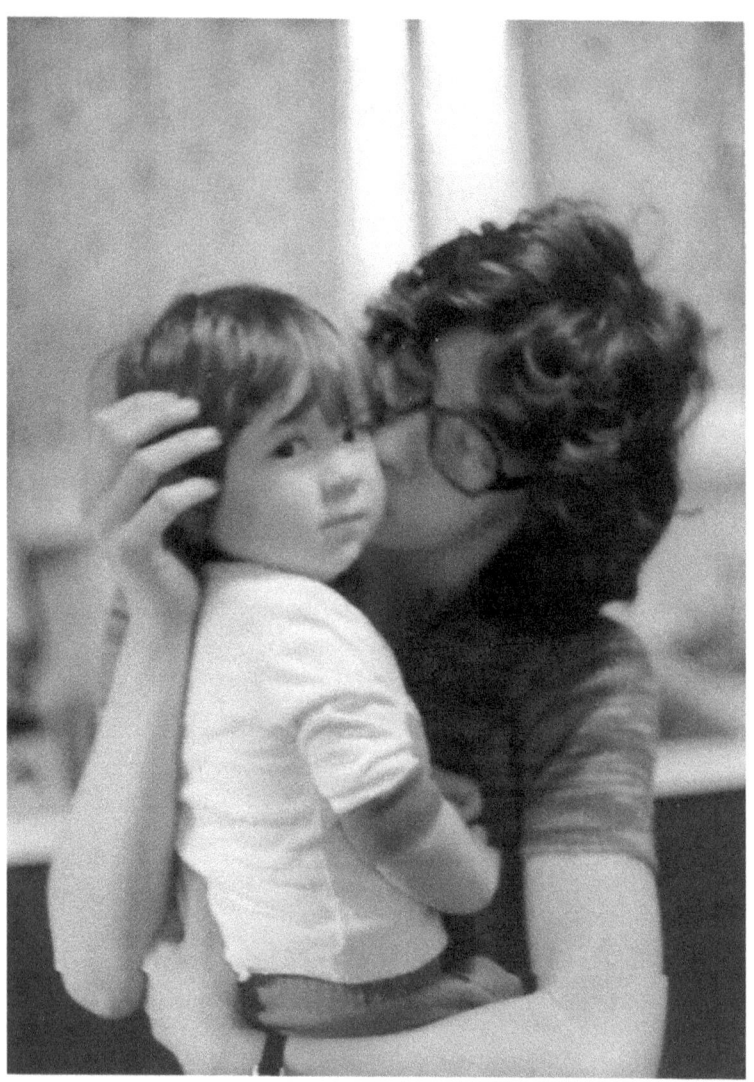

"And when the night is cloudy,
there is still a light that shines on me.
Shine until tomorrow,
let it be.
I wake up to the sound of music.
Mother Mary comes to me,
speaking words of wisdom,
let it be."
- The Beatles

A Foreword by Dr. Karen Cowden Dahl, Sandra's Daughter

A mother lost...

"On my honor, I will try to serve God and my country, to help people at all times, and to live by the Girl Scout Law." We recited this Girl Scout Promise every Tuesday at our Brownie Girl Scout meetings. I had wanted to be a Girl Scout for many years, mostly because my older brother was a boy scout. To me, scouting meant badges, camping, and friends. I was so determined to be a scout that, when I was around three, my mother humored me and made a merit badge using a leather tag from an old pair of blue jeans. It was not until first grade that I finally became a Brownie Girl Scout. As a young Brownie, the Girl Scout Promise did not harbor deep meaning. The promise was just a phrase to memorize. As I entered second grade, those words became bigger and more important. I realized that "to help people at all times" would become my life's direction.

Brownies met after school at the troop leader's house. She lived a couple blocks south of me. I usually walked home after the meeting. One of the Brownie moms drove some of the other girls and me from my school to the Brownie meeting on Tuesday, November 12th, 1985. I looked out the window as the car drove past my house to our meeting. A knot formed in my gut when I saw the ambulance, yet I said nothing. On some level, I knew the worst had happened. Maybe my brain was protecting me from the inevitable. Or maybe, at seven years old, I was too young to process why there was an ambulance at my house. Maybe I needed two more hours to be a kid before my life was forever broken.

We had fun at our Brownies meeting. When it was time to leave, I saw my grandmother parked in front of the troop leader's house. As I climbed into the tan pickup, I knew why my grandma was there. I don't remember Grandma's words, but she broke the news to me that my mother died that morning. Grandma drove to her sister's house. Our world began to crumble. We were at my Great Aunt Grace's for an eternity. I wanted my dad, but I didn't know where he was. I knew I was alone without either of my parents. I assumed he was making arrangements at the funeral home. When he finally arrived, there was a pain in his rusted eyes I had never seen before. His voice was low and soft. My heart breaks each time I picture his face that day. For as much pain as I was feeling at seven years old, I knew he was feeling far more.

Each morning, I would kiss my mom goodbye before school. That morning, I had forgotten. I was probably in a hurry or trying to avoid the image of my mom suffering. In her final days, my mom could only lie in bed, unable to eat, talk, play, or be a mother. My mom's life force was replaced by The Tumor. She was the victim of a frontal lobe tumor of the brain, known as a "glioma." The frontal lobes have many functions including motor skills, forming memories, empathy, personality, creativity, and judgment. The cancer directly impacted my mom's personality and behaviors, so we named the intruder in our house, "The Tumor." We watched my mom suffer and deteriorate for months. Cancer is a sadistic fascist that seizes control of its victim. It slowly destroys the host's body, mind, and even humanity. The despot then wields its cruelty on the family and friends by gnawing at their emotions, finances, and hope. I watched this terrorist target my family since I was two years old; I knew its tricks and what to expect. Since death was circling my house and peering in through the windows my whole life, it wasn't scary or unfamiliar. My dad sat down with me in his oversized yellow chair a short time preceding my mother's death to tell me that she would die. It was surreal, but not sad or scary. My mom was sick most of my life. I was not surprised to learn she was dying. I did not want my mom to continue suffering. She was in constant pain. For months, her actions and behaviors changed as The Tumor gained power. My mom was already gone before that Tuesday in November when she died. So, when my dad told me she was dying, I was ready for her pain to end, and for the asshole Tumor to stop torturing her. Brownies had taught me to always help others, but on that day on my dad's lap, I was powerless to help my mom or my family. Only death could ease my mom's suffering.

The next few days after my mom's death were a blur. My dad's family arrived from Wisconsin. Neighbors brought us food. My brother and I missed a few days of school. We had a rosary for my mom, visitation at the funeral home, and a Catholic funeral. The days were engulfed in sadness, yet it felt too busy to be sad. I thought I should be seen crying, but I was not crying. In the twisted reality I existed in, The Tumor was still winning. Instead of feeling sadness, The Tumor delighted in seeing me relieved. At seven, I was relieved that my mom was no longer in constant pain. However, that pain metastasized from my mother's body and spread to my dad and my brother. My brother was devastated. He locked himself in the bathroom for hours. I assumed that everyone would expect a similar sadness from me, but that is not how I felt.

Instead of sadness, I always felt lucky for the time I had with my mom. She was diagnosed with a brain tumor when I was two. My very first memories were of my mom in the hospital and her recovering from brain surgery following her cancer diagnosis in 1981. I was pouring myself a cup of milk one day and spilled. I proceeded to clean it up with a blue washcloth. I was so proud of my two-year-old self, I ran to my mom's room to tell her of my achievement. She was lying in bed in a dark room sleeping. I was not supposed to bother her when she was sleeping, but I wanted to tell her what an excellent job I did. Mom had stitches on her head and my brother convinced me to call her Frankenstein. I did not understand. She didn't look like Frankenstein to me. She was always beautiful. These were my first memories. I have no memories of my mom before she had cancer. For me, instead of sadness, I felt relief that my mom's suffering was over, and I felt blessed that my mom successfully fought off The Tumor for four years so that I would have a few happy memories of childhood with her.

During my mom's brief remission from 1981-1985, my mom fit in a lifetime of joy and ambition. I remember going to Girl Scout camp with my mom. We went to a fair and the Balloon Fiesta. My mom taught me to read. We had tea parties and played games. I helped Mom with her macrame and I watched her Jazzercise classes. She was an amazing soul, a pillar of strength, and truly used her life to serve God, her country, and others. At the same time that Mom was filling our lives with joy, my mother's tyrannical roommate (The Tumor) was plotting a comeback.

Despite The Tumor, my mother was braver and stronger than she ever believed. My mom moved twice across the country, the first time just weeks after having brain surgery. Following the trauma of being a cancer patient, my mom wanted to help others so she began taking graduate classes to become a therapist. She found time for fun activities. Mom did the best she could to be a wonderful wife and mother while pursuing personal goals. Finally, she wrote her own memoir. My mom began her writing slowly by jotting her experiences on notecards. As her writing progressed, my mom filled spiral notebooks and began to type up her book on a typewriter. My dad even built my mom a desk at our house in Wisconsin so she could have a dedicated writing space.

Writing became a form of therapy for my mother. As a female patient in the early 1980s, my mom felt alone, unheard, and scared. She also hoped that her experiences would provide comfort to other patients living with illness. Mom was an empath, mother, wife, nurse, sister, daughter, friend, artist, and dreamer who instilled in me her DNA, willpower, and intellect. Mom inspired me to help cancer patients, too. I have spent the last twenty-six years researching cancer. Now I am keeping my Girls Scout Promise to help others by amplifying my mom's voice and sharing her story so that she may have an indelible impact on American healthcare. The Tumor took her from this earth at the age of thirty-four, but her words will live for eternity.

I'll begin with an introduction of my mother, then let her own words take it from there. After, I'll conclude her story and provide context for what has been done in cancer research.

Help people at all times! Fight and win the war on cancer! Girl power!

My Mother's Story

Sandra Ann Garcia was born to Beatrice and Tobias Garcia on December 1st, 1950. She had three younger siblings in a strict Hispanic household in Albuquerque, NM speaking mostly Spanish. She started school at a small Catholic school. At first, school was difficult as my mom was disciplined for not speaking English. While she quickly learned English in school, her early struggles negatively impacted her confidence. She nevertheless graduated high school and was the first in her family to earn a college degree. In June 1971, my mom married my dad, Robert "Bob" Cowden. My parents both attended the University of New Mexico. My mom was a nursing student and my dad was in pharmacy school. After they completed college, my parents started their family. My brother, Ken, was born in 1975 and I was born three years later in 1978. My mom worked part-time as a nurse. We were a typical nuclear American family until January of 1981 when our world crumbled.

In January, The Tumor invaded and altered my mom and our

family in every way. As she will tell you, Mom suffered physically and emotionally. Despite suffering the trauma of a cancer diagnosis, my mother set on a path to use her pain to serve other patients. My mom dedicated the next phase of her life to healing, surviving, helping others, and continuing to raise her family. However, her journey was shorter than expected. My mother's life ended three weeks shy of her thirty-fifth birthday. She accomplished her goals of being a nurse, a wife, and a mother. Being a cancer patient gave my mom new aspirations. While she was a patient fighting for her life, she did not receive sufficient support from the medical community. Doctors were often sexist, failed to communicate with compassion, or were even cruel. My mom saw a niche in the healthcare system that needed to be filled. She wanted to comfort suffering patients and assist them in coping with trauma. Mom began graduate studies in counseling. As a nurse, she saw many sick patients, but being a patient changed her view on healthcare and how patients are treated. In her memoir, my mom provided a detailed account of her journey as a cancer patient, her trauma, and a glimpse into the challenges cancer patients face.

Please note, my mother's writings predate much of our knowledge of the etiology of cancer. As of this book's publication, we know that cancer is caused by mutation or aberrant expression of genes that results in abnormal cells in our body reproducing uncontrollably. So, while I did not alter my mother's story, I do provide scientifically accurate information as footnotes herein, especially where my mother speculates correlative causes of cancer. I also provide minor clarifications to my mother's text in brackets to help readers understand who a person is or their connection to my mother. Text in parentheses is directly transcribed from my mother's writing. My mother's memoir was written in English and only edited minimally for grammar and spelling for the reader's benefit.

A Posthumous Memoir
by Sandra Cowden

CHAPTER 1

"Congratulations, it's great to be alive." Jerry J. startled me as he almost jumped over the nurses' station counter to hug me. I'm a thirty-year-old registered nurse, working at a VA hospital in Tomah, Wisconsin. The above happened when Jerry came to me complaining that the drugs he was on just seemed to be too much, leaving him sleepy much of the time during the day.

I said, "Know what you mean." Jerry looked at me unbelievingly as if to say, "You, drugs?" So, I began to tell him my story. I said, "I was in the hospital last January."

He said, "Do you mind if I ask you why?"

I said, "Not at all." I began my saga.

January 4th, 1981 did not start out much differently than any other morning that I worked. It was a cold, dark Sunday morning when the alarm aroused me at 5:30 a.m. Although I was rushing to get dressed, I was only going through the motions as I really didn't look forward to work. At the time, I was working at Lovelace-Bataan's OB-GYN unit. Actually, I liked working with maternity patients: teaching breastfeeding, helping new mothers bond with their new babies, teaching postpartum care and newborn care, and just holding a baby now and then, since my children were growing up. I was also getting some limited labor and delivery experience, and I was eager to learn. What I didn't like was the prima-donna attitudes of the doctors working on that unit. An example of this was the time Dr. Meinhart told me that an infected C-section patient only had a hematoma (the effusion of blood into the surrounding tissue). While working at the University of New Mexico (UNM) hospital I had seen so many infected C-section incisions, that I wondered if the doctors washed their hands before surgery. So, I often left work with unrelieved anger brewing.

After driving across town (not a drive I enjoyed), traffic was heavy. A twenty-minute drive took thirty minutes. I arrived at the hospital at approximately 6:30. It was still dark, and I parked in my usual spot close to the hospital so I wouldn't have to walk far in the cold. After running to the hospital (I always ran when it was cold), I went to the women's locker room and changed into scrubs and took report at 6:45. This Sunday was different in that no one was scheduled for labor and delivery except for Barbara who was "on call." A patient came in, so I called Barbara who said, "If all you've got is a patient in labor, I'm not coming in." Not being as assertive as I would be now and also being inexperienced in labor and delivery—not knowing how rapidly a laboring patient's condition could change—I did not insist that she come in.

After taking report, I went to check the patient in labor and all of the other patients on the floor. While checking on the laboring patient, I stayed to start the IV, put the fetal monitor on her, and take her vital signs. I knew my services were needed there as Geri (a new RN) had not yet been certified to start IVs by herself. After I reassured the patient and called the doctor, I called the supervisor for more help, but she could not or would not provide any so Geri, and I had to manage as best as we could.

Everything seemed to be going all right for a while, but I seemed to have trouble keeping a good heartbeat with the monitor, so I called Geri to try and adjust the monitor. In the meantime, I did a vaginal exam, and the patient was progressing quite rapidly. I called the doctor when the patient was dilated about 8cm (10 is fully dilated), as I didn't have that much labor and delivery experience. These particular doctors preferred to be called when the baby was "crowning," when the head could be seen in the vagina.

Dr. Meinhart arrived around 9:50 a.m. and asked if I called anesthesia. I said, "No, but I'll call them right away." Then he began raving and ranting about the fact that anesthesia should have been called by now. (I think if doctors could see how they looked when they ranted and raved, they would cease the temper tantrums and talk civilly to people). Anyway, I called anesthesia and when I reached them, I asked Dr. Meinhart if he would like them to come. He took the phone and told the anesthesiologist (who happened to be the head of anesthesiology) that he did not need him. I believe he wanted to make an impression that he could handle it himself as at this point an anesthesiologist was required to be in the room when a baby was delivered. But it was Sunday, and he would not come except in an emergency.

As it turned out, it was an emergency, and at 10:03 we delivered a slightly depressed baby. Dr. Meinhart began yelling again that I had not called anesthesia before he had arrived, failing to acknowledge the fact that he had refused their services. As Geri and Dr. Meinhart tried to suction the baby, I ran to call the pediatrician. The telephone operator got the message mixed up and called the obstetrician instead. I ran back to the phone and told her who to call and she started to apologize, at which point I hung up because she was wasting more precious time.

Dr. Spencer came on the scene at about 10:50, asked when the baby was born, and was of course angry when I told him. He left for a while, then came back with the supervisors and asked why it had taken so long to get ahold of him. I said, "I told the operator to call the pediatrician, instead she called the obstetrician. I called her back to say that it was the pediatrician I wanted. She began to apologize profusely, so I hung up."

Dr. Spencer asked me whether or not the baby had been suctioned at the perineum. I said, "No, only after delivery." He said, "Next time hand them one of these (a mucus trap) and they'll have to suction at the perineum." A mucous trap is a little bottle with two tubes attached, one to suck on and one to suction the baby with. I told Debra, the nursery nurse, to take the baby to the nursery immediately.

During this episode, I was feeling a mixture of conflicting emotions—anger at Dr. Meinhart for not accepting his responsibility over the situation, anger at the nursing office for not providing more experienced help, sympathy, concern, and love for the poor baby who had suffered as a result, and an increasing anxiety over what was to come of all this.

I felt like crying when I went to the conference room to write my notes and eat my lunch, but it was a relief to sit for a while. There was an extra tray, but I just picked at it. Any hunger I had was dissipated by the morning's events. So, I spent my lunch hour writing my notes, carefully documenting Dr. Meinhart's refusal for anesthesia services, the operator's mistake, and all the other necessary data.

I rose from my chair to put my tray back on the rack and the next thing I remember is being flat on my back in the emergency room. My first thought was, "What on earth am I doing here?" Eilene Hansen, the day supervisor kept saying she would call my husband Bob. She was an absent-minded redhead who I no longer had confidence in after this morning's events. She probably couldn't even handle a phone call, I thought to myself.

In the meantime, the emergency room doctor said, "I'm Dr. Barber, the emergency room doctor. From what I can gather you had a grand mal seizure. Well, you were incontinent." I was so embarrassed, as the only people I knew there were the people I worked with. He could have had more tact, I thought. I felt kind of alone with no one to give me support.

The doctor proceeded to ask the usual questions to find out if I was oriented. He asked what day it was, where I was, etc. I was proud of myself when I said January 4th, 1981—not 1980. I thought I might trip up because of the New Year. They felt I was on drugs and did a toxicology study in addition to the routine labs. I felt incensed by the fact that they would think I was on drugs, but I know if I protested it would increase their suspicions. How simple it would have been if it had only been drugs! With all that had happened, I didn't have a lot of time for thinking, but I began to worry that Bob hadn't come yet. Apparently, Eilene Hansen had trouble contacting him, but she failed to inform me of this. So, she left me in a state of nervous anticipation, since by this time I had begun to realize that they were not going to release me. Dr. Barber said he was calling in a neurologist, Dr. Smith. Then he proceeded to tell me that he was a good neurologist. It's so reassuring when they add a comment like that, and almost as an afterthought.

After doing a chest x-ray and electrocardiogram, I was sent up to a double room, which I did not like. By this time, I was becoming aware of sensations that had been erased by the brief spell of unconsciousness. Suddenly, I became aware that I had a severe headache. The patient in the next bed had oxygen flowing, which sounded like thunder to me. Bob had somehow found me in the corridor while they were wheeling me to my room. I extended my arm when I saw him; I was glad to see him.

The thoughts that ran through my mind at this time ran something like this, "Oh no, epilepsy! At my age?? Epilepsy means driving restrictions, etc." I had treasured my independence especially since my parents had been so restrictive and driving was a symbol of independence. The other thing that concerned me was that it might be some sort of stress-related seizure as a result of this morning's events.

By the time I had settled into the bed, all I could think about was getting medication for the pain and something for the nausea, since now, in addition to the headache, I was experiencing nausea and vomiting. I also wanted a private room. I kept repeating these requests to Bob and the nurses, despite the fact that I know that neurologists are often reluctant to provide medication because they fear it will mask symptoms of the disease or injury. Bob kept reassuring me and telling me to be patient.

The nurses were taking my vital signs and neuro signs fairly often, although I don't remember how often. The nurse was a young dark-haired girl, with her hair tied back because it was so long. I recognized her as the wife of one of the doctors on staff. She did introduce herself to me. Then she began to ask me questions. Did I have an aura before the seizure? For the third time, I told somebody that I'd never had a seizure before and didn't know what an aura was like, but I hadn't felt anything before or during the seizure. I felt infantilized by the bed pads, although I knew they were for my own protection. Also, the flashing of the flashlight in my eyes was irritating because it increased the intensity of my headache.

Two hours later I was transferred to a nice suite that they usually reserved for VIPs. The suite had brown carpeting, a chest of drawers, and a window on the left with brown plaid curtains. These were the "ritzy" rooms of the hospital. I told Bob I would like to make love here.

I also got medication about this time. Earlier in the shift, a young attractive male nurse entered and said, "My name is Lenny and I'm your nurse tonight." He gave me the injection in the derriere. I thought I would be embarrassed, and somehow, I wasn't. I told him I was concerned that, because of the hospital rules, they [would] not let my children in. He told me not to worry. My defenses were somewhat dulled by the seizure, and I made flirty gestures toward him, something I had never done in my life!

Sometime that afternoon, Dr. Smith was in and told us what he planned to do all the while looking at Bob. He proposed to do a CAT scan, computerized axial topography, or a fancy X-ray machine, which produces computerized pictures of the body's organs, much like the computerized pictures taken at state fairs.[1] First a picture is taken without dye, then they insert an IV with radiopaque dye to get a better picture. He also intended to do a sleep-deprived electro-encephalogram (EEG). In this test, they keep you awake all night, wash your hair the night before, and apply electrodes on your head in the morning. The electrodes are then connected to a machine which records and measures the brain waves on a two-inch strip of graph paper, much like an EKG. They probably use the same machine, only they attach the electrodes to the head instead of the chest. Lastly, he wanted to do a spinal tap. With that, he opened a can of worms with me. In nursing school, I had seen a traumatic spinal tap on a child and ever since had fainted upon seeing a spinal tap, except when holding a child for a tap, and then I didn't look.

---

1 When this text was written in the early 1980s, CT scans were a newer and innovative technology. Computerized pictures at the state fair were state of the art.

Dr. Smith was a short man, with black curly hair and somewhat lacking in self-assurance. He spoke softly and rapidly, not pausing for questions and sometimes stuttering with a word. Nevertheless, I had to interrupt him in order to express my concern over the said procedures. I had to tell him that I always fainted when I saw a spinal tap.

And I said, "Dr. Smith, I'm allergic to IVP dye used in CAT scans."

He nonchalantly said, "We can give you medication before the CAT scan and you can't faint when you're lying down." Again, I was faced with a chauvinistic male doctor, and still at that point in my life, I was too inhibited to tell him what I thought of his unconcern. My anger over egotistic, narcissistic doctors was surmounting but didn't explode until I got to La Crosse. In the meantime, Dr. Smith continued to address Bob, and not me, throughout my hospitalization.

Later in the evening, some of the people of the fourth floor OB-GYN staff, the floor on which I had been working, came in to visit. I began to inquire about the baby that we had delivered that morning. Whenever anyone came in from the unit that evening, I asked how he was. My underlying but primary concern was the baby's welfare. When the girls assured me he was doing well, I breathed a sigh of relief. I had to keep verifying the facts. Even though I felt Dr. Meinhart was responsible for the poor delivery, I felt a sense of guilt too. I was still angry at Dr. Meinhart, so I didn't mind telling them how I felt. I kept saying, "Dr. Meinhart's an ass, Dr. Meinhart's an ass." I remember thinking that normally I'd never had said such a thing, but I didn't care. I raised a few eyebrows in the room.

That night I was given a sedative, which I didn't refuse because I was so nervous, I thought I needed it. I was also started on Dilantin (an anticonvulsant) and Valium. As sensitive to drugs as I am, the next few days were fuzzy. I awoke the next morning in a cloudy sedative mist only to receive an injection of Decadron and Benadryl to prevent any allergic reaction. So, on Monday, January 5th, I had an EEG and CAT scan, both of which I vaguely remember because it seemed more like a dream than reality. I didn't mind the CAT scan or EEG at all since I vaguely remember them.

That afternoon was dark, cloudy, and gloomy when Dr. Smith sauntered into the room. He walked so slowly that it seemed he took one step forward and two steps back. I guess he would rather not deliver the gloomy news, gloomy as the afternoon. When he finally walked around to the left side of the bed where I could see him better.

He took a deep breath and said, "We found something. We won't need that thing." He was pointing to the spinal tap tray.

I felt relieved that a spinal tap was unnecessary, but my heart began to pound and beat faster, and I asked, "What's wrong?" not really sure I really wanted to know.

Avoiding the question, he said, "Well, we need more information; we plan to do an arteriogram." An arteriogram is a test in which a catheter is inserted into an artery then fed up into the brain or other body organ that they may wish to study and followed on a scope. It requires the use of intravenous radiopaque dye.

Thoughts raced through my mind as I remembered the four-year-old boy who died while I was caring for him as a result of a cardiac catheterization, whose catheter wandered away and traveled by the bloodstream into the brain. And they wanted to insert one into my brain! Needless to say, it is a painful test.

Because Dr. Smith was vague and indefinite, my terror grew. Bob had already left when the nurse brought in the permit for the arteriogram that evening. The permit said that one in two hundred have a complication of a blood clot to the leg or the brain, which in the case of the brain would mean immediate death. (Sometimes, knowing a little is bad). I told the nurse I wanted to talk to the doctor. In the meantime, I panicked because I considered one in two hundred rather shallow odds, especially with my life. While the nurse was gone, I called my best friend Katie and told her that I thought that one in two hundred odds were rather shallow and how frightened I was especially after seeing the four-year-old die after a similar procedure. She said they were, but not any more so than childbirth. That relieved my anxiety a teeny bit, but enough to get me to sign the permit. I still wanted to talk to the doctor.

When the nurse came back, she said that Dr. Smith was not on call and that I would have to talk with Dr. Melrose (the interventional radiologist). Dr. Melrose called my room directly. I told him I was concerned about the one in two hundred odds of a blood clot to the leg or brain. He said, "What do you want me to do about it?" He didn't improve the odds or reassure me that 99.5% of the time nothing happens. He just got defensive and said that I could go to the Mayo Clinic if I wanted and that they would tell me the same thing.

The nurse on the evening shift had more concern for my anxieties [and] had me talk to a patient who had an arteriogram the day before. He said they'd stick a catheter in your groin, then you'd feel a warm feeling in your head and that's all there was to it. Simple for someone who doesn't know what can happen, even though they explained the risks. Many people do not understand medical terminology and do not ask for a simpler explanation for fear of sounding dumb.

I was, again, sedated the next morning. However, I don't remember the injection as I probably received it before I had awakened. I vaguely remember being on a stretcher and being wheeled to the cath lab with Bob holding my hand. The cath lab was cold, probably refrigerated, and all I had on was a sheet. The stark white and silver of the steel also contributed to the chilling environment. The antiseptic was enough to drive the most stoic person away. The cath lab was a small white room, with white walls, with a long narrow table that shone like sterling. An enormous white, bright round movable light, very much like a dentist's, except much bigger hung overhead. The effect was much like a dentist's office also. Momentarily, I wondered how they got a very large person on such a narrow table. There were a lot of people gloved, gowned, and masked, so any modesty I had was wiped out. Actually, I felt very humiliated, but didn't have long to concern myself with that, because of what was about to happen.

The screen the images projected on was on the far side of the room, above my head, so I couldn't see what was going on. But from experience, it's much like a small TV set except the picture is in black and white and comes out in lighter and darker dots, like a computerized image, except moving.

I was shaking under the sheet while the girl was shaving my groin. Fortunately, she left the top half of the sheet on me, or I might have turned into an ice cube. She was a dark-haired, dark-skinned girl who had gloved and gowned but had not put on the OR cap or mask yet. I was glad I could see one person in order to relieve how detached of a situation it was. She also held my hand during the procedure. Bob was there but I guess they didn't let him get too close to me, but he was watching the results on the screen. I was still shaking while she was shaving me, and I didn't know whether it was from cold or fright. But she was friendly and soothing, even though I was shaking like a leaf.

The stick of the catheter hurt but that was the least of it. The arteriogram was AWFUL. The feeling was hot, not warm. It felt like I was on fire.

I thought I was going blind and kept yelling, "Stop this, I'm going blind, I'm going blind," over and again. Of course, they didn't stop it and both the doctors and nurses just kept telling me to be still. The girl who shaved me held me to keep me still. The humiliation was heightened because I felt like I was in an auditorium with hundreds of people watching. But that was the least of my problems now. I don't think I was aware of the embarrassment until later.

That afternoon, Dr. Golden (neurosurgeon) came into my room, introduced himself, and said there was a need for a biopsy, that they would release me later, but that I was to come back next Monday. I really don't remember this, but it must have happened. Either these memories were suppressed or overpowered by this morning's emotions. I don't think I was ready to accept the fact that I had a tumor; even though they never said it, there were hints, like the ominous word "biopsy."

CHAPTER 2

Fortunately, they let me spend the next three days with my family. I'm not sure I enjoyed them; I was numb. It was like I was in a fog or a bad dream. I really thought, "Oh! This is not really happening; I'll wake up and this nightmare will be over." I don't remember a lot about those three days. My speculation is that I was in shock. At home, I would get as close as possible to Bob and shake uncontrollably, as if his life force could transfer from him to me. The closeness and love [were] the only good thing[s] that resulted from this crisis. It was the silver lining behind the cloud.

It was a chilly but warmer than usual January 11th when I once again entered the hospital. Although I was still frightened, I [was as] resistant as I had been for a previous operation, knowing the seriousness of the diagnosis. I knew it had to be done. Mom came to get the kids while Bob took me to the hospital. We arrived at Lovelace-Bataan[2] in the early afternoon, perhaps a good time because my friends at work came to visit. One of the "benefits" of the illness was being the center of attention. Geri Hauser, a new graduate, and the nurse who had helped me with the delivery four days ago, dropped by in the early afternoon to visit. Geri was [a] tall, dishwater blonde girl who believed in metaphysical powers and was a "strict nutrition nut" often eating goat cheese and unleavened rye. I liked Geri a lot but didn't like eating with her

---

[2] Lovelace-Bataan was a medical center in Albuquerque, NM. It is now Lovelace Medical Center.

because of the odor of her food. Geri had some trouble adjusting to the real world of nursing, and I had been the one to help her out. For what Geri lacked in clinical skills, she made up for in her warmth and intelligence. So eventually, I knew she'd come along. For a moment I wished I was in her shoes, instead of in this bed. How I hated hospital beds, especially the sheets. They always chaffed my skin. And I always scraped my elbows on the sanitized sheets and received sheet burns. Then I realized that I'd never want to be a new graduate again.

Geri came to me and said, "Go ahead and let it all out." So, I did. I cried and cried until I could cry no more, while Geri hugged me. This, somehow, seemed to irritate Bob, and after she left, he said, "I have four people to worry about; you only have yourself." I suspect he wanted me to reach out to him and that he wished that he was the one that provided such comfort. I was so needy at this point. I was reaching out to anyone who was open and available. I would have thought that would have taken some of the pressure off him.

Some of the terror of entering the hospital was squelched by the fact that friends visited. All I could think about was asking to see the kids. One of my greatest fears was that I'd never see them again. Mom and Dad brought the kids that evening and I hugged them and kissed them and told them that I loved them. They were loud and jumped on the bed, but I was not embarrassed by their antics. But Mom was and she suggested they leave after a short time.

Dad, of course, had to kiss my forehead and remind me of his relatively minor eye and skin surgery. He has always been a bit of a hypochondriac who could contract almost any disease whether it was possible or not. Ken, my son, became worried that he had caused my illness, because in one of his angrier moments he had wished me dead. Five-year-olds have trouble distinguishing between fantasy and reality and their own imagined power. I asked Bob to ask Sally, the next-door neighbor, to take him to see the priest to see if he could explain to Ken that it was not his fault that I got sick; it just happened that way.

Ken told me the next night, "I know you're going to be all right

Mom, the priest said so." It gladdened my heart to hear him say that. I learned later that the whole parish had offered a mass for me.

I had met Melanie Brooks when working on the OB-GYN unit at staff meetings. She was the nurse counselor for the hospital. She came in that evening to see how I was doing. She helped me a lot by just being there. She came just about every day, and we became friends.

The evening nurse brought in the operative permit, which said, "Right Craniotomy and Frozen Section of Tumor." Isn't it odd how the first place the word tumor is used is on the operative permit? Also, I was told I was to only have a biopsy. It might not make much difference to the lay public—the difference in the use of words—but to me, a biopsy is the taking of a small sample of tissue and a much shorter procedure. Obviously, the procedure had not been properly explained, so I refused to sign the permit until I could speak to the doctor. I had concerns and questions I wanted to be explained to me, like exactly what they were going to do. Also, the thought of them shaving my head and leaving me bald bothered me enormously. I was not worried so much as whether or not the tumor was malignant (cancerous), but whether I'd make it through the surgery or end up paralyzed. God had never let me down, so I had a special clairvoyance that the tumor was not malignant.

As I am usually sensitive to drugs, my anxiety must have been monumental for although I received Valium, Dilantin, and a sleeper, I could not sleep. A black heavy-set nurse came in to sit with me awhile, but she talked constantly of food and then went to get some. I was N.P.O. (nothing by mouth). Then she had the gall to eat in front of me. I guess she thought it was better than leaving me alone to imagine the worst. I must have finally slept, although it was way past midnight.

The next day was January 12th, and the drugs must still have been working because I awoke in a haze. I was aware that Bob was in the room and that we spoke, but much of the memories of this day were erased by the drug Ativan, a drug in the Thorazine family given to me purposely to make me forget.[3]

Dr. Golden came in about 9 a.m., it seems. I had lots of questions. But he answered them, unabashed by my asking them. I wanted to know where the tumor was, how long an operation it was, what effect the operation might have on me, and why the only symptoms were only a few severe headaches and the seizure. I also wondered what the purpose of the frontal lobe of the brain was.[4] I still dreaded the shaving of my head and asked if it was necessary to shave it all. He said since it was a frontal tumor, he would only have about three inches in front shaved. He said, "Well, I suppose we could shave about this much," making an imaginary measurement on my head.

Dr. Golden began to answer my questions. He said he'd do a bifrontal incision and that they'd do a frozen section.[5] He could not answer how long the operation would take; that depended on the involvement or what effects it might have on me since that also depended on how much involvement there was. He also didn't have an explanation as to why I had so few symptoms. I had told him that although I had occasional severe headaches, that they were usually relieved by vaporizers, decongestants, and aspirin or an occasional Darvocet. He said the only explanation was that the frontal lobe is a silent area of the brain and that little is known about its function, except that it is concerned with thoughts and feelings. He also said I'd have to spend a day or so in the ICU. My fear increased and I thought, "Oh, my God," and I began to realize the seriousness of the diagnosis. But I succumbed to this feeling of knowing that he must know what he's doing. Besides, I liked him. He had charm.

He was the first doctor that was personable and took the time to talk to me. We talked [for] about an hour and a half, and the subject diverted to Wisconsin, when he found out that Bob was from Wisconsin. He informed us that he had done his residency there, at

---

3   Ativan is a drug used to manage stress and anxiety in patients. Ativan was likely prescribed for anxiety. Ativan use can result in memory loss.

4   Sandra's tumor was located in the frontal lobe of the brain.

5   A frozen section is taken to the pathology lab where the pathologist (doctor that will make the cancer diagnosis) will stain the tumor section and determine the type and stage disease. In Sandra's case, the pathologist would determine the type of cancer (tumor) and the severity of the cancer.

the Gundersen Clinic in La Crosse.[6] The topics we discussed were diversified. And if it was his intention to put me somewhat at ease before the operation, he accomplished that. As he was about to leave, he asked me if I'd like something to make me forget this day. I agreed. I did not want to remember all of the frightening details.

Bob said that I screamed with pain from the pre-op shot that contained the Ativan. I'm usually calm about taking injections. Bob said the nurse dreaded giving the shot, so it must be a real painful shot, though I remember nothing of it. Bob said that I had said that it hurt all the way down my leg. The operation began at about 11 a.m. and lasted until about 3 p.m. It was a four-hour operation, and the drug was effective since it did produce an amnesiac state for about twelve hours.

The operation, I know from experience, is not pretty nor is any operation. But brain surgery is especially difficult to look at. After shaving the portion of the head and making the incision (which probably looked quite sickening since the skin on my head would have hung over my face because of the type of incision it was), they take a drill and drill three little holes in the head, then connect the holes with another incision making a triangle. Then, they leave one side of the triangle intact, so they have a flap that is easy to close back up. When they are done, they replace the "burr holes" with special metal burr hole caps.

The next thing I remember was waking up in the ICU. I was hooked up to an IV that was connected to an IVAC machine. An IVAC machine helps keep track of the rate that IV fluid is infused.

As the waves of consciousness submerged and rose, I slowly became aware of my surroundings. There was a beige-colored curtain around me, and the nurses' station was to my left. I felt that my head was bandaged, and although I couldn't see myself, I imagined I looked somewhat like a mummy. I was aware of some pain but not near as much as with abdominal surgery. However, they must have wanted to keep me quiet as they were giving me Morphine IV push every two hours. When I asked Dr. Golden,

---

6 La Crosse, Wisconsin is a small city about 40 miles from where Bob grew up.

later, why there was so little pain, he said that the brain interprets pain for all the other parts of the body except itself.[7]

My first memories upon emerging from unconsciousness were set in a thick, cloudy mist-like setting. Everything was in slow motion and a chubby nurse in a blue and brown plaid-trimmed scrub suit that the hospital had just purchased for them floated in. She removed the EKG leads from my chest and then washed off the sticky gel and probably gave me a bed bath. I asked for another blanket.

She said, "Of course."

I said, "Thank you."

I don't know if I looked surprised or what, but she said, "We give all our patients good care." Maybe I was surprised because when I had Karen[8], I didn't get any of my requests.

I spent the next twenty-four hours in the ICU fluctuating from sleep to wakefulness. On the evening of January 14th, I was transferred to a private room on another floor. I was moved between the third and fifth floors, so I can't say which floor I was on now. The window was on my left and I could tell it was dusk by the setting sun.

A rather large, grandmotherly type nurse walked into the room. I was transferred from the stretcher to the bed, just scooting across the stretcher to the bed.

As soon as I was settled, the nurse said, "When do you want the Foley catheter out?"

I said, "As soon as possible."

This answer surprised her, and she responded with, "Are you sure? Then you'll have to walk to the bathroom."

I said, "I'll walk." I was eager to regain my independence and could never understand why anyone would want a Foley just because they were too lazy to walk to the bathroom. I also began to feel that people were beginning to see me as an invalid. One day,

---

[7] The statement about the brain and pain is simple but correct. The brain does not feel pain because it doesn't have the right receptors (nociceptors). Pain receptors in other tissues (parts of the body) send signals to the brain that translate into pain.

[8] Karen is Sandra's daughter.

Katie's mom brought me a bed jacket.[9] I accepted graciously, but never used it and returned it as soon as I was able.

The first time getting up, though, did cause some lightheadedness, but the nurse and Bob were there to help. I was just beginning to realize just how often Bob was there. And once the anesthetics and narcotics wore off, I was also beginning to become more aware of my surroundings. I also began to appreciate the shocking reality and gravity of the situation.

I felt a great need to reach out for help and since I could do little more than walk around the bed, I developed an obsession to make phone calls. I guess, in a way, I felt an instinctive urge to "settle my affairs." Carol, my sister, and I had never had a good relationship. We were born two years apart and the sibling rivalry was great. But I wanted to talk to her and let her know what was going on. Dad gave me her number but, despite this, I managed to get the wrong number. Bob kept asking me if I dialed right but did not prevent me from dialing. This was the first indication that I could not remember things and I was becoming increasingly upset.

I must have called Carol three or four times before I got through. I informed her that I was in the hospital and [had] just had brain surgery. She asked me many questions, many of which I couldn't answer. She asked me who my doctor was and had to be sure I was getting the best care. I assured her that I was receiving the best care and that the chief of staff had been in the operating room.

Dr. Smith came in at about 5:30 p.m. He started pacing back and forth. Bob was in the room. Dr. Smith said, "You have an astrocytoma Stage II. It's benign. It's definitely not malignant but it is potentially malignant. I discussed it with your husband and we both agreed that you should have the treatments for insurance only."[10] At the time, I agreed, but even then when I was mostly alert, I didn't realize

---

9 A bed jacket is a robe.

10 While it is true that an astrocytoma Stage II may be benign on a pathologist's report, the median survival in 2023 is five to eight years. Benign is a clinical description; it does not mean that the tumor is not deadly or severe. I point this out because I do not believe my mom understood this, or she thought that benign is equated with curable. However, this lack of understanding provided needed hope for my mom.

that he was talking about radiation treatments. What I felt was a burning anger at being treated like a child. He and my husband decided what was good for me without even consulting me.

About that time Dr. Golden walked in and Dr. Smith said, "I-I was just telling them...we thought Mrs. Cowden should have the treatments." He always seemed a little unsure of himself around Dr. Golden. Dr. Golden took a step backward and explained that they had taken out most of the tumor, but they had to leave some behind because they couldn't cross the midline or corpus callosum or some loss of function could occur. A psychiatrist later told me that they didn't like to cross the corpus callosum because it would affect the learning center of the brain. They also performed surgery on the right side of the brain because I am right-handed and the right side of the brain controls the left side of the body and if I lost any function, they would rather it be on the left side. (The left side of the brain controls the right side of the body.)[11]

Dr. Golden asked me if I had any concerns. I told him, "I keep dropping things and can't even remember what I'm going to say next." I told him that earlier that day at lunch, I even missed my mouth. He seemed amused that I should be so overly concerned about this but reassured me that it would pass in about a month.

Supper was served at about six o'clock. I had trouble getting the food into my mouth without dropping it. Ted and Alice and Bob and Dave were in my room (close friends of ours). I'd start to say something, then forget mid-sentence. I found this new difficulty extremely frustrating.

Dave recognized this and with a sense of humor he said, "You're not any more forgetful than I am, and I haven't just had brain surgery."

Days weren't too bad and left little time for thinking. I had plenty of company especially at the change of shifts when the 4S (a floor I worked on), and pharmacy people visited. But nights were terrible.

---

[11] Brain surgery is complicated and how a tumor is removed and how much tumor is removed depends on the individual case. Without access to Sandra's imaging or patient records, we cannot validate the reason that complete resection of Sandra's tumor was not possible.

I'd wake up, not always sure of where I was and once I realized where [I was], a pervasive anxiety would return. I did not know what to expect, so I could not deal with it alone.

When I did wake up alone and frightened, I'd often call Betty Height, the night nurse on 4S. She would either come up or talk to me on the phone until I was able to go back to sleep. Nights on 4S were usually very quiet, but once in a while they were busy, and Betty couldn't talk, so I'd have to find someone else who would talk to me. Though I don't remember, Katie, my best friend, said I called her at 3 a.m. I learned that this October when I went to visit her after her baby was born. I apologized profusely, but she said, "It's okay. You needed me then and I knew you wouldn't always need me at 3 a.m. and I couldn't be there in the daytime, so I was glad to be there for you at night."

When I finally got over the nighttime jitteries, I would sleep until morning. The next morning, bright and early, the maid brought in towels and fresh bedding. Bob was already there when I awoke. Breakfast came and he helped get me comfortable in order to eat. I had chosen pancakes as I dislike cereals and eggs, but as I've never been a big breakfast eater I just picked at it.

Bob filled the tub and helped me in. It was a good thing he was there because after a few minutes, I swooned as I was getting into the tub and could have fallen and hurt myself. The syncope was caused by orthostatic hypotension, caused by lying in bed and the warm moist air in the bathroom. I was grateful, however, that I had a tub in the room and did not have far to go.

Still, I felt guilty because Bob was doing everything for me. I told him, "You know the nurses are here for that."

He said, "I want to do it." I felt he was getting exhausted and was also struggling with the feeling that people were treating me like an invalid. I didn't know it until later, but Bob was also watching that my blood pressure did not go too high, as I normally run a very low blood pressure, but was running a higher blood pressure since the operation. He did not want it to get too high for me, as one of the signs of intracranial pressure is a rise in blood pressure and a decreased heart rate. After my bath, I realized that I had a red, red papular rash all over my body. The pruritus that accompanied the rash was very annoying.[12]

The doctors came in about 10 a.m. and, as uncomfortable as I was, I told them that I had a nasty rash and threw up my gown to show them. Bob was embarrassed and he teased the doctors by saying, "What'd you do to her? She used to be a nice quiet girl. Must have changed her personality."

The doctors laughed and Dr. Golden said, "Yeah, we went in there and changed her personality." It was a big joke to them, but I felt my identity and privacy were already stripped and I had nothing left to hide. However, I laughed, too. Any joke was worth breaking the melodramatic mood.

The doctors decided I was allergic to Dilantin, so Dr. Smith switched me to Tegretol. He also ordered Benadryl, a drug to relieve the itching, and Caladryl lotion to apply topically, also to relieve the itching. Between the scratching, [the] application of Caladryl lotion, [and] the nurses' interruption for vital signs or medications, I mostly slept. Bob said that I slept through some people's visits. My wakeful period seemed to be evening and night. Perhaps it was then that my anxiety was highest.

Jennifer, a girl whom I had worked with on 4S and a little bit on labor and delivery came to see me that morning. She had resigned because of the way the OB-GYN doctors treated nurses. I mentioned to her that I thought Bob was getting exhausted and I didn't think he should be helping me with my bath.

She said, "Well if it was him, you'd want to do it, wouldn't you." I replied that I didn't think I could, but I saw her point.

I must have been complaining about "that awful hospital food" because Katie and Dave brought me a huge pepperoni and green chile pizza, my favorite. By this time my appetite [had] fully returned, in fact, I was famished after twenty-four hours NPO, and then that icky hospital food. I nearly ate the whole pizza by myself and thoroughly enjoyed it. Later that night when Katie and Dave left, Katie told Bob that she had never seen me eat so much.

By January 15th, I was beginning to get bored. After my walking,

---

12 Pruritus is the itchy feeling that makes one want to scratch.

I would read a little, a very little. *Hanta Yo* was about Indians, and I had always been fascinated by the Native American culture, but in this book, the boys changed names every time they accomplished a new stage in life, so it was very hard to follow. I wanted to stick with it though and read about four hundred pages out of nine hundred before giving it up. In the many hours of the day, I breathed into the spirometer, slept a lot, and occasionally asked for a pain pill.

It had been twelve days since I had worked so besides getting bored, I began to miss the babies in the nursery. I woke up at about 3 p.m. I knew the evening shift was beginning, tried to read, waited about an hour and called the newborn nursery. The evening nurse Andrea answered. I told her how I missed the babies and made the ridiculous request that she bring up one of the new babies for me to hold. Only I didn't consider it ridiculous at the time. I'm glad Andrea had a sense of humor. She did not mock or deride me or read me the riot act; she just chuckled and said, "Sure, I'll see you later."

I began thinking that a year ago I would have thought the idea of my having a brain tumor ridiculous. So, in some of those long, endless hours I just tried to capitulate about what had happened. What I didn't realize was that I was sleeping too much in the day and not enough at night and that caused the wakeful nights, and everything is scarier at night. The other thing I didn't realize was that I was being overdosed on Tegretol. The blood levels had not yet peaked while I was in the hospital.

That evening after report, Andrea came in. Of course, she didn't bring any babies with her, but she filled me in on the unit gossip. There had been problems between labor and delivery and postpartum. It was a territory battle. Both personnel were expected to cover both places, but each felt an ownership of their separate places, and that made relationships strained. That's why I liked working in the newborn nursery; they were not involved and all the better for it. After talking shop, she left, but by that time Bob was back.

Knowing that there were periods in the day when I was becoming bored, as I was more awake and the book *Hanta Yo* that I had borrowed from Betty Height only put me to sleep, Bob brought me a backgammon game and Katie taught me how to play. Jennifer had also brought me a mini-scrabble game, one good for use in the hospital or in the car as the pieces stuck to the game board. Other than playing with Katie I never got the chance to play games as when the visitors came, we had a lot to talk about.

As more people visited, the room began to look like a funeral parlor as it filled with flowers. At the time, I didn't notice; I don't even think it occurred to me that it looked like a funeral parlor. I just appreciated their thoughtfulness and enjoyed them. Even the girl from the cath lab sent a card and flowers, even after I made a fool out of myself there. But it made me wonder whether it was all the benign the procedure they said it to be. What had other people been like there?

Another unexpected surprise was that two girls from the ER had given me a card and flowers. I didn't even know them. The card read, "A friend of Bob's is a friend of ours."

I continued to have an obsession to make telephone calls, so in the breaks between visitors, doctors, and nurses, I continued to call people. I called Trina Jakes, my old head nurse at Bernalillo County Medical Center.[13]

The next day must have been January 17th. I had trouble keeping track of the right date as the nights ran into days as I had no calendar, and the drugs had affected my perceptions.

Melanie [the nurse counselor] was always there for me. I could always rely on her to come in every day. I guess it was her job. But it was more than that; we eventually became friends. Mostly, Melanie just sat in my room quietly, just listening if I wanted to talk. I am surprised by how much I opened up to her. She'd come into my room and say with a real enthusiasm to see me, "Hi, how are you feeling?"

"It hurts some but not as bad as my abdominal surgery did." In fact, it hardly hurt at all compared to that.

"I saw Bob out in the hall. He's really holding up well for all that you two have been through. How's everything else going?"

---

[13] Bernalillo County Medical Center is now the University of New Mexico Hospital.

"Well, I was really angry when Dr. Meinhart tried to blame me for not having anesthesia there when that baby was born, but I was unable to express it."

"It's over now and you know you'll never change them (OB-GYN doctors). How does Anne (the head nurse) feel about your work?"

"Oh, she thinks it's good but that I should be more assertive."

"How do you feel about that?"

"I think so too but I have to take my time to accomplish it."

"Sure."

"You know that I was able to express my anger to Dr. Spencer but not Dr. Meinhart. Dr. Spencer came onto the unit one day yelling about why we hadn't gotten his patient to surgery yet. I told him that she had arrived five minutes before from the ER and she was on her way now. Later he apologized."

"Don't worry too much about them. Anne has been trying to change them since she got here but has not had much success."

We both chuckled. Anne had been trying to get these particular doctors to improve and update their practice. She had ordered a new infant resuscitator, which they got mad about because they didn't know how to use it. Only one out of the four was receptive to change.

I was very interested in her career as a nurse counselor, as I had always been more interested in psychology than nursing but never changed my major because my mother had said not to waste her money.

"Melanie, I'd like to go to graduate school but I'm wondering if I'd get in because I only have a 2.8 or 2.9 grade point average."

"After you've been out of school for five years, that doesn't matter much anymore."

"I'd like to do something like you're doing and have thought about applying to the Guidance and Counseling program."

"No, don't do that. Stay in nursing. You'll get more money that way."

"You mean get my masters in psychiatric nursing."

"Yes."

"Thanks."

"You bet. Goodbye, I'll see you tomorrow." She turned to go. But I wasn't alone for long. The 4S staff came regularly. They brought flowers and a nightgown. Brenda, the unit secretary, brought two small shakers of Avon powder. I thought that was especially nice of her since she often became annoyed when I checked her orders or translated Spanish for some of the doctors or nursing assistants. Brenda seemed to enjoy speaking Spanish in order to keep secrets from people.

My days were spent with meals, walks, breathing into an incentive spirometer, a gadget with a blue hose and four clear tubes with blue balls in it. The object of the game is to blow into it and breathe deeply enough to [make] all four balls go up and down. It helps to expand the lungs after a general anesthetic. I had told Dr. Golden to get one ordered for me because I had sinus problems and tended to get congested easily.

The days began to seem interminable as fewer people began to come. Also, the Valium created a cloudy world and I had not yet felt the effect of having to have radiation treatments. I was also beginning to be drugged by the Tegretol.

The rash seemed to take its time in leaving and I continued to use the Caladryl lotion, but I was still depending on the Benadryl to keep me reasonably comfortable. I was more alert in the evening when the drugs had started to wear off and just before they dosed me again.

Just about sunset on the evening of January 16th, around six or seven o'clock, Bob brought me some Chinese food. The dinner he ordered included fried lettuce, chicken chow mein, pork fried rice, and barbequed ribs. It was all so scrumptious. I was also disappointed this evening. Mom and Dad didn't show up, but that's not what upset me. They didn't bring the kids and since my illness, I had developed an obsessive need to see them, as at this point in time, I didn't know what to expect. It might be the last time I saw them.

Bob said he could see my point, but he could also see how tired and harassed they might feel after taking on two active children and bringing them to the hospital every night, especially at their age.

So, when he left that night, I felt a little sad and lonely. Every time I was alone at night and uneasiness overtook me, the kind of feeling one has just about the time something scary in a movie is about to happen. Fortunately, the evening nurse entered and said, "My name is Nancy, you seem familiar. Could you have possibly worked at UNM hospital?"

"Yes, I worked on the post-partum about a year and a half ago."

"Well, it's a small world. I'll bet that's where I saw you. I had a premature baby girl two years ago. She's all right now."

"Well, then I must have seen you in the postpartum unit or in the nursery. We used to take the mothers over to see the babies especially, if the mother had a C-section." We chatted a little more about each other's children, the problems her daughter had, and only a little about me. But she listened to my feelings and that was important. It was also refreshing to get my mind off myself.

I had another visitor that night, a quite unexpected one. Winifred Lewis had been in the army and as a result, acted like a tough army sergeant and acted like one on her unit. Actually, she worked in Labor and Delivery, but the nursery, L&D [Labor and Delivery], and the postpartum unit had to cooperate and help each other when one or the other was low on patients or help. She not only came off like a tough army sergeant, [but] she also looked like one. She was 5'6" and weighed two hundred pounds. I had been a little intimidated by this woman by her actions and gruff manner, but I was not the only one. Some of the other nurses, very good ones, were also intimidated by her, especially the ones who worked L&D regularly. Winifred and I had a sort of falling out. But we had gone to a workshop together and while I had visited with some of my UNM hospital friends. Winifred and some of the other Bataan nurses asked me to have lunch with them. I accepted. I had gotten the "pleasure" of sitting next to Winifred at the restaurant, something I had dreaded at first, but it turned out to be a very pleasant luncheon. We talked. She learned that I was an intelligent person with good ideas, and I learned that she had a heart after all. She even went to the extent to tell Bob that although I was a quiet person that I was all right.

But still, somehow, I didn't expect her to remember when I was sick. Maybe, I got that feeling when another nurse on the unit died. People went to visit her during working hours, but nobody thought to give flowers or some other gift. I even blamed myself for not making another visit or making the suggestion that the unit get her a gift, as I had been thinking about it.

The conversation with Winifred turned out to be quite interesting though. We discussed doctors, working conditions, other staff members, and my tumor. I expressed my hopes and dreams for the future, and she told me a little of her many adventures around the world.

I ate my supper, washed up, and walked around awhile. At about seven o'clock, Trina Jakes (my former head nurse) arrived. She brought me a dish garden. It was really quite an attractive dish garden. The dish was about a two-foot planter with many kinds of plants, including an asparagus fern, philodendron, some kind of ivy, plus other varieties for which I don't know their name. Trina was rather amusing. She kept repeating how she had bought that instead of one type of plant because "with so many plants, at least one ought to survive." Guess she had heard about my "purple thumb" or maybe I mentioned my "success" with plants. She would be glad to know that, in Wisconsin, the planter is doing just fine.[14]

Actually, she wouldn't have had to bring a gift to cheer me up. Trina was so verbose, enthusiastic, and ebullient that it was hard to be gloomy around her. And of course, she caught me up on what the old crew at UNM hospital had been up to the last year and a half. Paula had moved on to [the] newborn nursery. Linda had graduated from UNM, gotten her BSN in Nursing, and had gone to work in an ICU in another hospital. I had already known that as I had become her friend and visited her when she got her condominium. (My kids drove her crazy). Linda was the funniest girl I ever knew. She would think up some good jokes and then tell them to our fresh C-section patients. They laughed so hard, they

---

14 Sandra lived in New Mexico when she was diagnosed with the brain tumor. A couple months later, she moved to Wisconsin where she began work on her memoir.

cried. Some of them said, "It only hurts when I laugh." She also talked of having triplets by C-section so she wouldn't have to go through labor three times. She didn't know what pain was.

Anyway, Trina went on telling me about the place. She said that everyone I knew there had left there on the evening shift except Kathy the nursing assistant, that they now had an evening secretary for four hours a night except for Saturday and Sunday, and that they [had] finally gotten more staff so they could do total patient care more comfortably. I said, "Real nice, everything gets better when I leave." However, I had no regrets about leaving as I did not get along with the night nurse and had no intention of working with her even on a different shift. Trina wished me good luck and gathered her purse and coat to leave. I said, "It's been nice talking to you. Tell anybody that's left, 'Hi.' Before you go, what about Sarah? What did she have and is she back at work?"

"She had a boy and she decided to stay home for a while. Better go before they throw me out." She giggled.

"Okay, thanks for coming, and thanks for the plant." She left and I felt pretty good about her visit.

But when the visitors and Bob had left, I'd start to feel apprehensive, but the nurses took care of that, at least for a while. They gave me Valium and sleeping pills, then I was snowed under at least until about 3 a.m. At 3 a.m., I'd wake up frightened. Then, I'd call Betty Height who was always willing to talk to me on the phone or come down and hold my hand if it was not busy. I always went back to sleep after talking to her.

I awakened just before dawn watching the pitch-black room slowly get lighter and lighter. As I was just sitting there with nothing to do, I reflected on all that had happened and decided that since I was getting so bored and feeling better, and that I had had enough of the hospital, that I would set out to convince Dr. Smith and Dr. Golden to release me. They entered at about 10 a.m. I began to request to go home, saying that I felt pretty good; that Bob still had a week of annual leave left that he took because of my illness. He would help me with the kids and the next week, I would ask my mom to stay with me. They were skeptical but said that as long as

I had help, they would let me go.

Dr. Smith instructed me to take one tablet of Tegretol four times a day. They made an appointment for me with Dr. Golden for the next week. Then they began talking about therapy again. At first, I hadn't realized they were talking about radiation therapy. I should have known, but the drugs dulled my intellect. At this time, I didn't realize all that radiation therapy entailed. Then Dr. Smith began talking about sending me to Los Alamos for the pi meson radiation treatments. It was the best radiation treatment available, but that's all he could tell me about it since he didn't even know if he could get me in. I don't know whether it was just because they had become fond of me or because I was one of "their" nurses, and a hospital becomes like a family, but they wanted me to have the best available treatment, especially Dr. Smith.

My tumor was not malignant, but potentially malignant. Tumors are classified into Stages I to IV, four being the worst. I had an astrocytoma Grade 2. Dr. Smith approached Bob and me with the idea of going to Los Alamos, and at the time we said we were interested in the program. So, he started the paperwork. Speaking about paperwork, the nurse began to fill out the discharge forms. On the afternoon of January 17th, I was released. It was an overcast and dull day, but to me it was beautiful. I was never so anxious to get home. Just getting in the car represented the first step of getting my freedom back.

CHAPTER 3

Getting home felt good. I had been anticipating seeing the kids regularly once again. I didn't know how awful I looked until they said, "Mom, you look like Frankenstein." And I guess I did. The suture line ran from about an inch off of the right side of my forehead, across the top of my head, and down the left side of my head for about an inch. I had a huge bump on the right side of my forehead, which was black and blue, and a smaller bump next to it, which was very sore. The bandage was off, but the sutures were still in place running the length of the suture line. Even though I knew that children are very candid and usually said the first thing that came to their minds, that remark hurt.

With sarcasm in his voice, Bob said, "Real nice, telling your mother that she looks like Frankenstein." Sometimes children's frankness is like throwing salt into an open wound.

How I had missed them though. I picked up Karen and gave her a big hug. I also gave Ken a big hug and kiss. Then they wanted a story, and they were still small enough for the three of us to fit in the big brown lounge chair. We settled down in the chair and I read a story. They begged for more, but recognizing that I was tired, Bob intervened and said, "That's enough, now let your mother rest." They complained a little, then went outside. Bob helped me out of the chair, and I went to the bedroom to lie down for a while.

While I was resting, I began to reflect on what effect my hospitalization had on them. Karen was so young and tiny and helpless in such a crisis. She was only two. And Ken, who could probably get along fine without me for a week, but I wondered how the guilt trip of having caused my illness had affected him. He had reassured me that he knew I was going to be fine because the priest said so, but still I wondered. He could be a handful if he wanted to be. I fell asleep thinking such thoughts.

When I awoke, I found Karen in bed with me. All she knew was that Mommy hadn't come home from work one day, and she wasn't about to let that happen again. She followed me everywhere after that! She had missed me. If I went to the bathroom and locked the door, she would sit outside the door whining and begging me to open the door.

Mom and Dad were still pretty frightened. They had to drop by that afternoon to see how I was doing. Bob fixed dinner that night, but Mom and Dad stayed for it not so much to eat dinner as to help Bob so that I wouldn't have to. It was nice to have someone to do the dishes. I hadn't realized just how much energy was required to just do dishes, even with a dishwasher. My energy had been zapped.

I had brought all my hospital paraphernalia with me, and our bedroom looked like a sick room. There was an apricot bed jacket Katie's mother had given me, my Caladryl lotion, the portable incentive spirometer, and the giraffe Alice gave me which I slept with in the hospital and would use at home for a while. Alice had said, "I always give my friends, kids or adults, a stuffed animal when they're sick." That was very thoughtful of her as many people do need "tender loving care," when they're sick.

Alice had a son five months older than my son who was quite different from my son, but we often discussed our various problems over the phone. Alice had come from New York, and I generally disliked New Yorkers, but Alice was different from the others. She did not come to New Mexico to take someone else's job nor did her husband. She and Ted came here for a more relaxed sort of life, turning down jobs of much higher salaries in New York. She was an open sort of person, very candid, yet never seemed to offend anyone by what she said.

The other articles included in my surroundings were a box of

Kleenex, my slippers, and a wastebasket close by. The book *Hanta Yo* was still there. I hadn't given up on it. The rest of the milieu consisted of the hospital kit that every patient receives. It includes a thermometer, an emesis basin, and a pitcher all backed in a wash basin. The beige telephone was also by my side.

The room was rather dark and depressing, especially with all the hospital objects around my bed. When we bought a queen-sized bed, I had bought a dark velvet red bedspread. I had bought another bedspread to make curtains out of. When the curtains were done, the room became darker. They were made of a heavy cotton and wool blend. The pattern consisted of a dark red background, matching the red in the bedspread, with white, and black stripes and little pink curly Q's. Since, at the time, I bought the bedspread Bob and I had been working the 3 to 11:30 shift and slept late in the morning, I had purposely bought the bedspread because the material was heavy, and it blocked out the early morning sunlight, and it was also cheaper than buying the heavy material in the first place.

I had taken my Tegretol and had gone to sleep at about 8 p.m. Unfortunately, the rest was short, and I was up by eleven. Bob was still watching television on the mossy green bag on the floor. I descended to the floor next to him and lay there literally shaking with fear. He would hold me tight, tell me to take a Valium. And when I returned from the kitchen after taking the Valium, I'd return and huddle next to him. We'd just lay in front of the television holding each other tight. Meanwhile, the Valium would take effect and I'd saunter back to bed and crawl in. After two or three hours I'd be awake and restless again. The first few nights after leaving the hospital were especially restless.

The next morning, the kids woke me bright and early Bob ushered them out and asked them to help fix breakfast. On school mornings the children received cold cereal and milk or instant oatmeal as Ken often had trouble getting ready on time. Going to kindergarten and getting up early was a new experience for him. On Saturdays or Sundays, we had a special treat of pancakes or French toast. Anyway, Bob got Ken off to school. Jack, the boy across the street, would often come get Ken for school.

Sometimes, at only five years old at the time, Ken would have doubts about my recovery, even though the priest had reassured him that I would be fine. He often would ask if I had to go back to the hospital. His uncertainty would increase as I made many trips to the hospital for blood tests.

Sally Taylor took over transporting the kids to school and did a great deal of babysitting. Other than Mom and Dad, she did the most for us in a bad situation. She is a buxom, selfless woman who helps people in times of need. She was very active in the church, helping to construct a playground for the children of Queen of Heaven School by organizing fundraising activities. She also got the whole congregation to pray for me when I had asked her to have the priest talk to Ken.

While Bob was feeding the kids, I rolled over and went to sleep for another hour. I woke up again at about nine, took care of the necessities, proceeded to the kitchen, and took my Tegretol. About an hour later I promptly vomited it. I had taken it with milk, but it wasn't enough. I called Dr. Smith and told him how terrible I'd been feeling. He said, "Did you eat anything with it?"

"Well, I took it with milk."

"Why don't you try taking it with food?"

"Okay, I'll do that." I hated how he patronized me and assumed it was my fault.

On Monday, my mom arrived as planned to help me out [during] my first week out of the hospital. She pulled into the driveway around 1 p.m. The doorbell rang [and] Bob answered it. He had his blue smock on ready to go to work. Mom said, "Hi Bob, how are you?"

Bob said, "Mean and ornery as ever." By this time Karen had heard Grandma and started yelling, "Grandma! Grandma! Grandma!" She was always excited to see her grandmother. Mom busied herself picking up toys, laundry, and other sundry tasks. I never had to tell her what to do. But she noticed my paleness and I could tell by the look in her eye that she was worried, but she didn't say anything.

Kindergarten was in session from 8:30 to 11 a.m. so that gave me some quiet time in the morning. Karen was never very noisy and now she had Grandma to entertain her. Both children loved to take their grandparents to their room to show them "all my toys." Grandparents love to spoil children, so they generally went and patiently waited while being entertained by the kid's display of all the many toys. Many were quite interesting, and Mom would usually steer their interest to those toys, like the train she gave Ken that would turn upside down [and] then change tracks. I'm sure Mom was fascinated by such toys that weren't around when she was a child; I know I was, especially when I was feeling better. And when they got tired of playing with the toys, Karen would turn on the television and watch Sesame Street or Mr. Rogers. But when Grandma was around, she didn't watch TV, because Grandma didn't come that often. Karen liked to help when someone said they had work to do. So, she followed Grandma around.

The day was exhausting. Although, I did little else but talk a little to Mom, sleep, stare blankly into the TV, and fall asleep again. I still had headaches and of course, there was some occasional incisional pain on the top of my head. I would take two Darvocets and go back to sleep.

Try as they might, children do not understand another's pain and an occasional scream, and sometimes not so occasional [screechings] would seep like a piercing bolt of lightning through my head, which explains why I had little patience with the children. Mom was there to help, but sometimes she was critical. When I said something to Ken, comparing him to Karen, she said, "Remember when you were little, you hated to be compared to someone else."

Although true, at times like these, I would become resentful. Didn't she know what I was going through? I was not yet ready to forgive. "How could she criticize?" I thought as I remembered my childhood. Me, my two sisters, and my brother were brought up in a strict Spanish-American and Catholic home. The methods of discipline were spanking, mostly by a belt, and very little provoked it. The most typical infractions to the rules were the normal sibling rivalry every family experiences. Occasionally, the fights would escalate to where adult supervision was needed, but we were never allowed to resolve our own conflicts. The home atmosphere was guarded and often frightening because my dad had a violent temper. The edict of the house was "Speak only when spoken to and children are seen and not heard." We had little experience making decisions, and then at eighteen, we were expected to go out and make decisions.

But I was grateful to have Mom there my first week out of the hospital since I couldn't have made it myself. So, I avoided arguments at all costs. Mom made lunch—soup, for she knew that was about all I could hold down. Again, I ate, took my Tegretol, and went to sleep.

I awoke about an hour later hot and itchy. I told Mom that I was going to take a shower. She said, "Are you sure you can do it?" Again, I felt that she was treating me like a baby, but I ignored it.

I said, "Yeah, I'll call for your help if I need it." I thought of how good a shower would feel. What I didn't think about was how the hot water might affect me and the orthostatic hypotension I might suffer from getting up suddenly. However, I was still itchy from the Dilantin rash, and a shower and a coat of Caladryl lotion would help keep me from scratching.

The bathroom was to the right of the bed. I gathered my underthings and a clean robe. To the right of the bed was the wood door, which led to our bathroom. The floor was a white linoleum with a pretty scrolled and grooved design, pretty but hard to clean. The white porcelain sink was on the right side of the bathroom and the toilet and shower stall were towards the left. The shower door was a hinged door with warbled glass to allow privacy. The walls of the shower and floor were tiled with solid peach-colored tile.

I slowly began to undress, avoiding looking at myself in the mirror and that was hard as the mirror was about 3x5 feet. I was still very self-conscious, well aware that I looked like Frankenstein. The bathroom began to steam until it looked like a Midwest fog, impenetrably thick with low visibility. But all I could think about was how good it would feel to soothe my aching muscles (from lying in bed) and itchy skin.

I opened the door to the shower stall [and] stepped down into the shower. There was a small step so the water shouldn't accumulate and run into the bathroom floor. I turned on the water, adjusting it to the hot side. I had closed the bathroom door but had not locked it.

As the prickle of the shower massage began to ease the tightness of my muscles, I became woozy and began to swoon. The room began to get dark, but I had the good sense to turn off the water and sit on the floor so as to not injure my head. I yelled, "Mom, help!" My voice must have weakened because, by the time she came, I felt better, so I told her just to stay close while I finished my shower. I concluded my shower without any further episodes of syncope.

That evening was pretty much the same as the evening before. Mom fixed supper, I went through the motions of eating, and Bob would clean up the dishes. Mom left just as we were eating so that she could go home and fix supper for her own family. What a load she must have been carrying even though she had taken a week off work.

Around 7 p.m., Katie and Dave came to visit, and it was always a pleasure to see them. We would talk [for] about fifteen minutes, then something would overtake me. I attempted without success to stay awake throughout their visit. Bob ended up entertaining them while I slept through half their visit. They noticed my inability to stay awake and left to "Let Sandy rest."

When they left, I again took my Tegretol, and back to bed I went. I was beginning to realize that I had probably been overdosed. The sleep I was getting was not normal sleep, but rather a sort of semi-consciousness that I could not control. I was so angry to be at the mercy of my doctor. But I had already called Dr. Smith twice that day and he was unrelenting in his opinion that this was the best medication, and it was the proper dosage. He said he had given more to little children. I asked Bob to talk to him in the morning, as Bob seemed to have a better rapport with him. Bob worked at Lovelace as a pharmacist at the time. I saw Dr. Smith as a male chauvinistic person, but I needed help and he seemed to heed Bob more. So began my battle with the doctors.

After I had been in bed awhile, I awoke to go to the bathroom. It's kind of humorous now, but at the time it was quite alarming.

The house was dark except for the small lamp Bob had over the TV. Still disoriented at night, I started down the black and eerie hallway. It was like a haunted house, yet I knew it was my own home. (Why I didn't turn on the light I don't know.) Then, I met little red and green men with pointed ears and tails. My first reaction was horror and dread, but then one of them turned out to be Katie and with speechless communication or telepathy I knew they were friendly and were there to help take me to the bathroom. I sat down in the middle of the hallway and began to cry. Bob heard my sobs, came down the hall, and asked what the matter was. All I could manage to say was that I couldn't find the bathroom. The real horror struck a few minutes later when I realized that I was awake, but this appeared to be a nightmare. Suddenly, I knew that I was hallucinating! Dreadfully, I wondered what the medication was doing to me.

Bob and I strolled down the hall arm in arm and lay together in the beanbag chair in front of the TV. We both knew I would not be able to sleep for a while. I did not watch much television. At times like this, I'd go through the refrains of a song in my head. The song was "Sometimes When We Touch," and the refrain ran "I'd like to hold you till I die; till we both break down and cry; I want to hold you till this fear in me subsides." And sometimes when we were holding each other close, the fear would subside and love would replace it, and Bob would ask, "Happy, baby?" I would reply "yes" because, at the moment, I was happy and had nothing to fear. At times like this, we were closer than we had ever been.

By the morning of January 20th, I knew something was definitely wrong. I dawdled over the milk and toast for what seemed like an eternity. It was hard to eat something when I was nauseated and while I took the Tegretol. In the endless time before breakfast, I tried to decide whether or not to take the Tegretol. Taking a drug that makes you sick is like trying to take poison. I pondered my dilemma. If I didn't take it, the blood level of the Tegretol would drop and the doctor would say, "I told you so; you just have to get used to it." And if I did take it, I would continue to be sick, but I was obstinate in proving my point, so I took the pill.

By noon, I was extremely ill. In addition to vertigo, I perceived the pictures on the wall as climbing up and down. I also started vomiting. After heaving up the toast and milk, my stomach was empty, but that didn't register in my brain, and I continued retching. It was like I was on a roller coaster that I couldn't get off of. Weaving from one wall to the other, I made my way back to the bed to the bedside stand to the telephone. I called Dr. Smith and informed him that I had seen the pictures on the wall climbing up and down. He said, "What?" confused by what I was saying. As toxic as I was, I was probably not too coherent, but I persisted in getting my message across. I explained, "You know pictures—photographs—you have some on your wall, don't you? Well, they were going up and down, and I've been vomiting all morning long; please do something." He told me to come up to the hospital for a blood test.

I then called Bob and repeated the story to him. He said he'd meet us at the emergency room door. Then he asked me, "Will we need a wheelchair? I answered, "Oh, yes." Was I ever thankful Mom was there. I'd never been able to drive that day. Mom made arrangements for Bob's Aunt Audrey to take care of the kids. Audrey was there in a couple of minutes as she did not live far. Mom and I had put on our jackets to be ready when Audrey came. Just as we were about to leave, I vomited all over my jacket.

While I tried to clean up part of the mess, I overheard Audrey say, "I think she got out of the hospital too soon."

Mom said, "I think so."

I thought, "How could we (or the doctors for that matter) [have] known they would have overdosed me." Rather than waste any more time Mom threw her jacket around me and braved the cold.

Mom and I climbed into her green Buick. I didn't think I could make the trip; I lay across the back seat of the car loathing the stench and messiness. I then realized I had been diaphoretic and that mixed with the emesis created a most unpleasant feeling. However, the ride lulled me to sleep, and I was no longer aware of anything until we reached the hospital.

Bob and I discussed what Audrey said later. We came to the conclusion that further hospitalization would have served no further purpose. It would have happened just the same, the only benefit being that the lab people would have come to me to draw the blood. <u>The whole incident could have been avoided by the doctor listening to his patient.</u>

We arrived at the hospital twenty minutes later. Bob was waiting with a wheelchair. Not that I cared much about my appearance, but I was a sight to see. With the sutures still sticking out of my forehead, my pasty white complexion, [and] the oversized jacket, I looked like "Frankenstein" or like Bob later said, like a reject from a concentration camp. If there was any time through this whole series of events that I wanted to die, it was then. When I saw Bob, I started crying.

Holding on to Bob and Mom, I scooted into the wheelchair. While Mom went to park the car, Bob whisked me away into the elevator up to the third floor, where the lab was. The lab is located on the clinic side of the medical center. The elevators separate the clinic from the hospital. They have doors that open on both ends, so that you can go either way, depending on where you want to go. The lab was on the clinic side, so Bob pushed the appropriate button. He must have already had the elevator on hold for it was the quickest ride I'd ever had up there. I usually used the stairs. He also had picked up the lab slips from neurosciences (the name of the whole complex of neurosurgeons, neurologists, and auxiliary help). The lab technicians were already ready. They had me climb up on the red table covered with white paper sheets. Thankfully, there was a stool for me to use. I sat facing the other people that were there sitting in school-desk-like chairs. A bright, cheery, and young male technician gathered his equipment, pulled the curtain, and asked me how I was. I answered, "Terrible, can't you tell?" He shrugged his shoulders and went ahead with his business of tying the tourniquet around my upper arm, sticking the needle, and watching carefully as blood filled the vacutainer. Although injections never bother me much, venipunctures did. I always felt a slight nervous tension at the moment they held the needle next to my skin just before they pushed it in, only to be replaced by pain, but I always had to watch. I don't like surprises.

As he was putting on the Band-Aid, my mind wandered. I was thinking of how young this technician looked. I knew that when you hit thirty and the doctors, policemen, and other working people begin to look like kids, you are getting old. Ann Landers said that.[15]

As we left, Bob commented that I should have been kinder. "After all," he said, "he might have thought this was feeling good for you." "I doubt it." I wasn't about to take a guilt trip for that.

I began to loathe the series of venipunctures that began because they couldn't get a proper therapeutic level of Tegretol. It took two days to get results, so mostly to pacify me and relieve the already toxic symptoms, Dr. Smith lowered the Tegretol dose to one tablet three times a day.

The hallucinations stopped but I was still sleeping twenty out of twenty-four hours a day and walking around like a zombie. Bob said, "My God, you just had brain surgery, you're supposed to be tired." But I didn't buy that and called my girlfriend Cher whose mother had taken anticonvulsants for many years.

I asked Cher, "Was your mother tired a lot?"

"Yes."

"No, but she laid down every afternoon for a nap."

"Well, I've been sleeping twenty out of twenty-four hours a day and I'm getting worried."

"But Sandra, you just had brain surgery."

I continued to snooze much of the time. Mom helped with the children, fixed meals, and did laundry. I know I was not the most exciting person at the time, but Mom began to discuss her problems and what she should do about them. She asked what she should do about Dad, whom she had become convinced was an alcoholic. I tried not to be irritable but replied rather curtly. I don't know if he was an alcoholic. I was not there often enough, and I don't know what you should do about your problems.

Two days later, Dr. Smith called. "I guess we poisoned you, ha ha!" he chuckled. I did not think it was at all funny. He informed me that my Tegretol level was twenty-one. Normal therapeutic level is from five to twelve. He lowered the Tegretol dose to one tablet twice a day.

---

15 Ann Landers was an advice columnist in the 20th century.

He also asked me to come in that morning and get another Tegretol level. The day happened to be Friday, January 22nd.

Again, Bob took me to the lab. It was a good thing he didn't start work until ten or eleven. This time, I was feeling somewhat better and took a look at the lab's waiting room which had a small lobby, about a quarter of the size of the neurosciences lobby I estimated. The vinyl and metal red and yellow chairs were the standard doctors' office chairs. The sun shone through the large picture window and gave off a bright glare, so I always sat with my back to the window. The technician came out and called my name, and I went in and sat in the desk-like chair while he drew my blood. The antiseptic smell of the inner office immediately hit my nose. The first time, I was so sick that I didn't pay attention to the minute details; this time, I did. The technician tied a yellow tourniquet around my arm, asked me to make a fist, and stuck a needle in my arm. The more often I got stuck, the more I dreaded venipunctures. As I always had to watch, I sat on the chair as they held the needle in the antecubital space [for] just enough time to increase the anxiety before inserting it into the vein. The bright red blood surged into the vacutainer, but the pain didn't stop until they withdrew the needle.

When I had talked to Dr. Smith earlier that day, he had asked me when my appointment with Dr. Golden was. I informed him that it was this coming Monday. He said, "Good, why don't we get another Tegretol level then? You can just pick up the slips when you're up here." I groaned but conceded.

In the hospital, I had asked Dr. Smith how long it would be before I could drive. He had said two weeks. Those were some of the longest two weeks of my life. Bob was patient in driving me places, mostly to and from the hospital for venipunctures. How I dreaded them!

On Monday, Bob took me up to the hospital at about 11 a.m. We had to go to the fifth floor of the clinic building where the neuroscience was located to get the slips for the venipuncture. We went through the same rigmarole at the lab. Only this time, a girl drew my blood.

The neuroscience lobby had a high counter with a desk behind it for the receptionists to use. It faces the elevator so that people can immediately tell the receptionists their business, without bothering the doctors or nurses. There's a nurses' station desk down the hall to the left and then shortly down to the right. The lobby is painted white, trimmed orange, [with] grey zigzag stripes up and down the walls; the modern décor that seems to be popular for doctors' offices and hospitals, but nobody likes. Four ceiling-to-floor columns dissected the room in six sections and created an illusion of privacy, where patients could hide their little secrets. The grey carpet hid any dirt that might have very well been drug in. The chairs were soft sofa chairs of various colors, so it wasn't too uncomfortable if you had to wait long, just annoying. I felt out of place here. Most of the clientele was over fifty. There were middle-aged people who had brought in one of their parents. There were people in wheelchairs, some with canes, and some who had obviously suffered a stroke.

Dr. Smith called that afternoon and said that the Tegretol level was fourteen. This time he lowered the dose to one tablet in the morning and one tablet in the evening.[16] He wanted another Tegretol level on Wednesday.

I was beginning to get depressed over the fact that they couldn't get a proper dose and getting downright tired of needle sticks, so I called Katie.

"Hi, Katie."

"Hi, Sandy. How are you doing?"

"Okay, I guess, except that I'm sleeping all the time and I'm so tired. The last Tegretol level was still high. It was fourteen and I'm getting tired of being stuck."

"Yeah, but you wouldn't want them to quit now until they get the right dosage."

"I know. But I'm beginning to feel like a pincushion. And I sure appreciate you listening to my gripes."

---

16 This was a confusing time for Sandra. She appears to reference two times where Tegretol levels were measured and dropped from 21 and 14. After each time, the medication was reduced.

The topic turned to kids and other things. Katie and I could talk for an hour sometimes, provided I didn't get interrupted by the kids. This time I was yawning soon after I called her and said goodbye earlier than usual as I had already been yawning throughout the call.

I wanted to get a nap before my friend Beverly came. With the dosage cut to only two a day, I had periods during the day when I felt better than others. I was also feeling good enough to care about my looks, so I called Beverly yesterday and asked her to go shopping with me for hats. I had remembered that Beverly always wore hats to work and always appeared very becoming. I called Trina, my former head nurse, and asked her if I could have Beverly's number. She said, "Sure." She then began a chatter of babbling conversation. Trina loved to talk. I worked with Beverly and Trina at the UNM hospital.

I had called Beverly and told her that I'd had brain surgery and would appreciate her taking me shopping for hats as I admired her taste in hats. I told her I always thought she looked very stylish. She was flattered by that and said she didn't mind driving me as I still couldn't drive.

So, I lay down to get a little nap before Beverly arrived. She was coming at 1 p.m. It was 11:30 and I figured I could sleep for thirty minutes before she came. Ken hadn't come home from school yet and Karen was watching Sesame Street.

At twelve, Mom woke me for lunch. I was still eating lightly and took a Compazine to keep the nausea away while Beverly and I shopped.

Beverly arrived at about 1 p.m. in a little red foreign sports car. I invited her in and introduced her to my mom. I said, "Beverly, this is my mom."

Mom said, "Mrs. Garcia," and extended her hand. I had always had a difficult time introducing my mother to other people.

I went into the bedroom to finish dressing while Beverly and Mom got to know each other. Simultaneously, Karen decided she wanted to go with us, saying, "I want to buy me hats, too." Mom persuaded her to stay home and "take care of Grandma."

As Beverly and I boarded her little car, she informed me that

Mom had told her that she hoped I didn't buy a cowboy hat, but she knew I probably would. As we drove to the shopping center on [that] mild, clear, and cool winter day we conversed about what had happened. Beverly asked, "How'd you find out you had a brain tumor?"

"Well, I was working one day, and the next thing I knew I was in a hospital bed. They told me I had a seizure."

"Did you have headaches or other symptoms?"

"I had some headaches, but I thought they were sinus headaches. I used a vaporizer, decongestants, and aspirin. Toward the end, they were more severe, and I was just beginning to think about getting help but I changed decongestants and slept in the beanbag chair because it seemed worse in the morning if I slept flat. These remedies helped, so I didn't pursue it further."

"You know, it's strange, you're the third person I've run into who's had a brain tumor. What kind was yours?"

"It was a frontal lobe tumor, astrocytoma, Stage II; they told me that it is potentially cancerous. They couldn't take it all out because of its location; something about the fact that they couldn't cross the midline."

"You know, that's the same kind of tumor my friend John had. He called me about three weeks ago and said had just gotten out of the hospital for that very reason. I wondered if brain tumors are becoming more prevalent, or if it's just a coincidence that I happened upon three people with brain tumors."

"Oh, it's probably just a coincidence, or maybe it's just that they're being detected earlier with all the fancy equipment they now have like the CAT scan. You must be feeling rather worried. It must be scary to know three people with brain tumors. How's your friend doing?"

"Fine." I got the feeling that she just did not want to discourage me.

As we drove on towards the shopping center, we continued to talk of other things such as how it was where we worked. She said she had transferred from post-partum to nursery and liked it much better. I told her that I had liked working at Lovelace-Bataan but did not like the doctors there who had such a God-complex, prima-donna attitude.

We went to the Coronado shopping center, stopping first at Goldwater's because it was closest to where we had parked. We saw some cap and scarf sets, but I told Beverly, "Let's look around for the best buy." So, we proceeded down to Dillard's and Sears. She would put hats on my head and either say, "That looks good on you, or let's try this one." That went on for a couple hours until, after lots of window shopping and browsing, we settled on three caps: a grey one with three white stripes; a dark blue one with purple, red, lavender, and white trim, and matching scarves; and a rather plain beige one. All the while I was trying on many hats, Beverly continued to comment on how it looked on me. I also bought a wool purple plaid "hunter's hat" with a rounded center and a two-inch flat brim. I also brought two tams: one rose-colored with a matching scarf, and the other a black velvet beret with a fake diamond pin. On our way out, we stopped at a Western shop, and I found a really nice hat. It was a cowboy hat, but it was made from 100% grey wool and trimmed with maroon-ribbed tape. The great thing about this shopping trip was that I only spent $48.75. We had hit the January clearance sales just right.

Dr. Smith wanted another Tegretol level on Saturday as he just could not believe the results that the lab had reported to him. I was very discouraged about this and told him I didn't believe it was a lab error because I was sleeping twenty out of twenty-four hours a day. But he insisted even though I could feel my voice breaking as I tried to hold back the tears. The Tegretol level came out eighteen this time.

Bob had understood how frustrated I felt and I was beginning to feel a little better since I was on just two tablets a day. He told me to dress up nice, that he had a surprise for me. After the trip to the hospital, he took me to El Seville, a hairstyling salon, where his friend Juan is the proprietor. I believe that Juan is the best hair stylist in Albuquerque.

I believed that Juan could do something with my hair, and I mentioned it to Dr. Golden when I had discussed how much hair they would shave off. Well, clever Juan pulled the back of my hair to the front and curled it under to create bangs, after which he of course had trimmed it. It looked much like Toni Tennille of Captain and Tennille.[17] I was very happy with the results, and what a boost to my ego.

That afternoon did wonders for my self-esteem. I looked better than I had in ages. I felt absolutely stunning and sexy and even more so when Bob surprised me and took me to the new Chinatown restaurant. We had lunch in the Moon Glow Lounge where the room is darkened for a romantic effect. There was entertainment, even in the middle of the day. There was a baby grand piano in the center of the room with a pianist who also sang. We chose a table close to the pianist. Bob ordered drinks while we browsed the menu. I told him I wanted what he had brought me in the hospital. It happened to be one of the luncheon specials. When the waiter came, he brought us a fine dish of chicken chow mein on top of fried lettuce and pork-fried rice. Of course, we always ordered a poo-poo plate, which consisted of egg rolls, barbecued pork and ribs, and deep-fat fried jumbo butterfly shrimp. After the bland and tasteless hospital food and the many soups I had because of severe nausea, the taste of the Chinese food tickled my taste buds. I savored every bite.

I was feeling a little giddy as I allowed myself two or three drinks. I was also more talkative than I usually was. As we drove home, we talked about what had happened, the good food, and the great job Juan had done with my hair. We wondered what Dr. Golden would think of Juan's talent. He had expressed the opinion that he thought nothing could be done about my hair.

We were both feeling good because of the drinks and also because we had missed each other so. Our desire and craving for each other had reached infinite heights. Two weeks was a long time. Once home, and the children still at Grandma's, we clung to each other, never wanting to be apart.

Our desires increased and we withdrew to the bedroom for a little afternoon delight. We made love carefully as the incision on my

---

17 Toni Tennille was half of the pop-singing duo Captain and Tennille from the 1970s with hits including "Love Will Keep Us Together" and "Muskrat Love."

forehead was still tender. It was beautiful, but still being drugged, I fell asleep and slipped into oblivion. The few minutes that I slept were more peaceful and relaxing than the many hours of dreamless sleep I had had the previous days.

I woke with a start and thought it hurt Bob's pride for a second or two, but we ended up laughing about it. Bob said, "Real nice, falling asleep while I'm making love to you." We continued to lay there and talk as I love to do after our lovemaking. After an hour or so, Bob decided he should go and get the kids, while I rested.

I was still in bed when he came back with the children. Since I was still impuissant, I allowed the children to play games on my bed for a while as I didn't have the energy to play their usual games. After they had enough time with me, Bob ushered them out, explaining that I still needed my rest.

I slept for another hour, then the telephone rang. It was Melanie, the nurse counselor. "How nice of her to still care, now that I'm out of the hospital," I thought. I don't know whether the hospital paid for her services outside the hospital. Probably not, but as a fringe benefit of the hospital, she was available to troubled employees free of charge. I might have known she would have called. While in the hospital, we had become good friends; I shared my hopes and dreams, realizing that my illness was like a chick breaking out of its shell. I was breaking the shell I had created and that had been created for me. I was ready to break loose and get control of my life, and Melanie patiently listened, rarely offering advice but always understanding and sometimes asking a question to make me think. I related my story of what had happened during the past week; how I felt about Dr. Smith always talking to Bob and treating me like a child. She empathized, and I always felt better after talking to her.

Bob made supper. Actually, he reheated the leftovers from lunch. Chinese restaurants usually give you more than enough food. They even offer "doggie bags." Actually, they put the food in little cartons for you to take home. We ate silently amidst the chitter-chatter of Ken and Karen. With supper over, Bob and I cleared the table and put the dishes in the dishwasher together. With my strength all washed out, I felt as if I had cement blocks tied to my arms and legs; they felt so heavy. So, in slow motion, I began to clear the table. I felt like Shields and Yarnell.[18]

The new morning sun broke the new day, and it was Sunday, a week since I'd been in the hospital. Bob and Mom both went back to work tomorrow, so I had to feel better. Since Mom hadn't come over the weekend, she and Dad arrived about suppertime. Again, Bob had supper on the table, but we welcomed them. Mom had brought roast beef cooked well done. She said she tried to cook it medium-rare like we like it but got carried away and it turned out well done again. Later, I puked up the roast beef that had been cooked well done. The aftertaste was repugnant. It tasted like putrid half-digested meat, and I could no longer eat roast beef for a long time.

Katie faithfully came just about every night. Dave no longer came with her, but I understood. She came to give me support. Dave had just recently lost his father to cancer, so he had a hard time facing illness and hospitals, especially [with] close friends like Bob and me. Katie mostly came to provide comfort and encourage me to get well. We said little, and I slept often, but she was there, and that was important. We have one of those rare relationships where we could talk for hours on the phone or say nothing and still be quite comfortable.

After she left, I had another restless night—the beginning of many to come. I don't think I slept a whole night through until sometime in May after the radiation treatments had been completed. So, maybe they were worth it if only for the psychological effect.

A crisp cold Monday morning arrived prematurely. It was my first week alone, so with trepidation I began to care for the children and myself again. Karen, I could count on to sleep until eight, sometimes nine. Bob got Ken up, fed him breakfast, and got him out of the door by 8:15 so he could be at school at 8:30. What I had to worry about was how he would act when he came back from school. He had had trouble getting ready on time, so I

---

18 Shields and Yarnell was a performing duo that had mime and dance numbers in the 1970s.

insisted he dress before he ate breakfast.

This morning, though, Sally thoughtfully again sent her son Jack to come and get Ken. Karen woke later. Bob had left for work, so I fed her breakfast although it seemed like I was taking one step forward and two steps back. I went through the same routine with my breakfast. After breakfast, we put our dishes in the sink and then went to watch TV. We would both lie down in the green bean bag chair. We watched Sesame Street and Mr. Rogers's Neighborhood and by the time it was 10:30, Karen would go to her room and play with her toys awhile or with her imaginary friends. I would get up from the beanbag chair and move to the couch to sleep there.

Ken returned from kindergarten at 11:30, bouncing through the door and announcing himself by yelling whatever kindergarten news he had that day. However, on that day I didn't hear him.

All of a sudden, I felt a jerking and shaking sensation and heard, "Mom, Mom, wake up, Mom." I heard him but could not respond. I kept thinking in my mind, "You've got to wake up. He'll be scared if you don't."

He keeps shaking me until I finally manage to say, "Just a minute, Ken, I'm having a hard time waking up." Until then, I couldn't even talk to reassure him that I was all right. Once again, I was riding the waves of semi-consciousness, almost making it to the top but just falling short and sinking into the depths of unconsciousness like a fallen surfer. I could tell by the panic in Ken's voice that he thought I was dead. So, I had struggled through the stages of unconsciousness, riding the waves from Theta to Alpha and finally back to Beta, or "the waking state." I then said, "I'm sorry Ken. I just couldn't wake up." I then asked him what he wanted and hugged him.

Ken had wanted a glass of milk, which I gave to him, and proceeded to make a simple lunch for the three of us.

I had an appointment with Dr. Golden at one that afternoon. Bob took an hour off work so he could take me. Dr. Golden kept Mondays open for appointments. I had sent the kids to Sally's after lunch and Bob arrived at about 11:45. We left at twelve since I had to have another Tegretol level done. Bob and I left not too concerned about the kids. Karen loved to play with Tammy, and

John entertained Ken so well. We said little as we drove down our little street, then out onto Comanche Road. As we merged into traffic, Bob asked how my morning had been. I told him about the incident with Ken.

We arrived at Lovelace Clinic at about 12:30. We stopped by the lab. I had "graduated" to sitting at the school-desk-like chair with an arm pulled over the front of the person separating the sticker from the stickee. With all the needle tracks, my arm was beginning to look like a junkie's arm.

With that over, we boarded the elevator and rode to the fifth floor. We told the receptionist who was facing the elevator who I was. Then she asked which doctor I wanted to see. I told her Dr. Golden. We waited for what seemed a long time. I was both anxious about the exam and bored, thumbing through pages of old magazines. When I got tired of that I would watch the other people with curiosity. A nurse came out and called a name. An old man with a cane stood up. She said, "Let me help you, Mr. Jones." Back to magazine staring, I stood up just to walk across the room to get another magazine and stretch my legs. This also helped relieve the anxiety. Bob smoked a couple of cigarettes, but I had never smoked and never wanted to. So, I disguised my pacing by getting more magazines.

Finally, a nurse came out to the front end of the lobby and called my name. We followed her down the hall. On the way, we met Dr. Golden. After we'd said "Hello," and all the other amenities, he raved about my hair.

First, he tugged it a little bit and asked, "Is it a wig?" He had answered his own question and said, "By gosh, it isn't." He was impressed by Juan's talent and said, "It sure is amazing what hairdressers can do these days."

The nurse led us into an examining room to the left of the nurses' station. The room had a wooden examining table, which I thought was unusual. There was a desk in the north corner of the room with a window right above it and a plant with a macramé hanger in the very corner of the room and a sink in the other corner opposite the table. There was an array of shiny silver-toned instruments on a tray, which was on a tray stand. Their display made me nervous.

In doctors' offices, since I was a child, whenever I saw equipment exposed in such a manner, I wondered what they intended to do with it.

The nurse had me sit up on the table. This one was a little homier because of the fact that it was made of wood. I sat up on the paper sheet looking around the room. Besides what I noticed upon entering the room, there were various degrees on the wall, which Bob was scrutinizing. We talked a little about the various degrees, and Bob seemed impressed and pleased that I had received such a good doctor.

Dr. Golden entered the room and immediately dispelled my nervousness. In a conversational tone, he asked how I was. He also asked if I had any questions and my first and only question was, "How long will it take for my hair to grow back?" He chuckled, touching his balding head, and said, "Well with me it seems forever." Then, he asked if I really believed what had happened. I shrugged my shoulders as I [was] still half hoping I would wake up from this crazy nightmare.

Still speaking in a friendly way, he conducted the first part of the examination without my being aware of what he was doing. In our chat, he had learned that I still had headaches, slight incisional pain, no seizure activity, no vision problems, excessive drowsiness, and no other neurological symptoms other than a small area on my forehead, which was numb. Still talking, he pulled the curtain, shut the light, and shined the flashlight into my eyes, instructing me to look at some object in the distance. He then told me to follow his finger with my eyes; then he held two fingers to the side of my head and asked me how many fingers I saw. He checked my reflexes with his little hammer. Everything seemed satisfactory, and he told me that I'd had no neurological deficit. He and Bob talked about several things. He anticipated Bob's next question and informed us that I'd live for decades. That took a load off my mind but did not cure the night shakes.

Dr. Golden then proceeded to remove the stitches on my forehead. It began to sting so I began to do my Lamaze breathing.[19]

---

[19] Lamaze breathing is a technique popularized in the 1950s to cope with pain during labor.

He said, "It doesn't hurt that much, does it?"

I said, "No, but I don't want it to hurt at all, and the breathing helps."

He then began discussing the radiation treatments. He asked me if I was interested in going to Los Alamos, New Mexico, where they have a new machine that emits a special ray called a pi meson. (Actually, the machine isn't so new; it's just in the last five years that it has been used, experimentally, for cancer therapy.) The machine is called a giant tandem Vandergraff particle accelerator. The pi meson ray is a radioactive ray that, reportedly, can kill a single cancer cell. That version may be a bit exaggerated, though, as some doctors become very excited about new developments in cancer therapy.

Dr. Smith said it could kill a single cell, while Dr. Golden said it was maybe ten percent better than regular radiation.

Dr. Golden asked me if I was interested in the program. I said I was, but I'd like to think about it. He sensed my reservations and sweetened the offer by saying that the residents were treated very well there; that it was like a holiday between treatments where the residents laughed, joked, and played games together. He said that the apartments provided for the residents were very nice and included color television. The residents were required to live in apartments close to the facility because the reactor was also used for various other purposes and sometimes broke down. So, they wanted the people available twenty-four hours a day. I asked if they would do treatments in the middle of the night. He said they might, but the nurse would call you. He said it's an impressive set of equipment; that it was eight city blocks long.

Still, Dr. Golden sensed my apprehension and said, "It's really quite nice; they treat you like a king there. I should live so good."

I was ambivalent about the whole affair. As I had never lived independently, I thought it would be exciting to live alone for a while. Then I thought, "What could be exciting about Los Alamos? It's just a small hick town with possibly one movie theater and one bowling alley." Also, the thought crossed my mind that Karen was too young to be separated from me for seven weeks. She was only two. On one hand, I felt that I should have the best treatments possible, and on the other, I knew it would be very hard on the family. One advantage was that there would be very little living expenses as the government subsidized the projects as research as the pi meson was still experimental.

Finally, Dr. Golden said, "You have a lot to think over. Why don't you have Bob let me know by the end of the week? Stop by the desk and make an appointment for next Monday, and we'll discuss it then. And remember, the pi meson is only this much more effective than ordinary radiation. (He used body language, putting his thumb and forefinger about a quarter inch apart.) It's very effective." I was mulling this through my head as we left the building. On our way out, we stopped by the appointment desk to make an appointment for the following Monday. We walked towards the pharmacy on our way out, and we met Melanie in the hallway near the pharmacy. She was so excited to see us and asked how I was doing.

But before I could answer, she raved about my hair saying, "Oh, I love your bangs. That's wonderful." Then she asked about the children. She was always concerned about them through this whole ordeal.

I told her they were well, and Bob said, "Mean and ornery, as ever." Then, we told her that Dr. Golden had recommended the Los Alamos facility for radiation.

She said, "Oh, you'll like it. I worked there and the people are all so nice."

Then, Bob came home that evening. We discussed the pros and cons of my going to Los Alamos. Bob said he would miss me greatly but whatever I decided was fine with him. He wanted me to make the decision so I suppose there would be no repercussions. I said, "Well I'll miss you all terribly, too, but I think I should have the best possible treatment." I was still influenced by the fear that was still within me.

Dr. Smith had finally lowered the dose of Tegretol to half a tablet twice a day and I was feeling better, that is, until about the middle of the week. I was still convinced it was the Tegretol. That had been a traumatic experience.

The next day, I came down with great fatigue and muscle aches and pains all over my body. Still thinking it was the medication, I called Bob to complain how rotten I was feeling, and having read in one of [Bob's] books, I was sure that it was the Tegretol because it said in rare instances Tegretol caused neuromuscular pain. I was sure I was one of those rare instances since it seemed everything was happening to me. Bob was not so willing to admit it was the medication this time. He was becoming weary of all my fluctuations between illness and health, but he continued to stick by me. He did, however, tell me he thought I had finally reached the proper dose. He said, "They can't go any lower or it would be ineffective. And I wouldn't want them to use any other anticonvulsants because the side effects of the remaining drugs are only worse." So, I waited out the duration (about a week). He told me that it was probably just the flu, as my defenses were so low.

When Bob came home that evening, he said that his friend Steve had the same symptoms that I had, so I accepted the fact that I caught the flu on top of being fresh out of the hospital and overdosed with Tegretol. But I guess when it rains, it pours. I also developed a vaginal itch, which I decided to ignore for the time being. If it lasted for more than a week, I would do something about it.

Bob had also talked with Dr. Golden, who informed him that [the] lab report on my tissue specimen had been sent to the pathologist, who examines the tissue for acceptance or rejection to the Los Alamos facility. He had told him that mine had been rejected, but he had submitted another specimen, just to be sure. He told Bob not to worry. Well, it seems that the second time around they found a very small amount of Stage III astrocytoma. So, I was accepted.

I had finally arrived at the decision that I would go to Los Alamos, so we had to tell the family that I was going to stay here while the rest of the family went to Wisconsin. In the meantime, my sister, Carol, had heard that you had to be on your deathbed to be admitted to Los Alamos. Carol is a medical technologist, working at St. Joseph's Hospital in Kansas City, at the time. She had asked one of the pathologists there about the Los Alamos facility and its program. He told her a very grave story and as we had told her that my prognosis was good; she became extremely upset, fearing that we had lied to her.

CHAPTER 4

On Thursday, Mom and Dad surprised us again as they often did the first three or four weeks after my surgery. I had to tell them our plans about moving and that I was going to go to Los Alamos. It was easier to talk to Mom than it was to Dad. So, when I gave the kids their bedtime snack, I invited Mom to help me. She came to the kitchen with me and said, "You can't pack all this stuff yourself, especially now."

I said, "You're right. Why don't you come over Saturday and help me pack?"

"Good idea," she said.

Unfortunately, after the episode of the flu, my physical problems were not over. On Wednesday, the vaginal itch had greatly exacerbated. Still, I was tired of doctors and decided to wait another day or two. Maybe a douche would help.

Anyway, it was nice that friends kept calling or coming by to give food or emotional support. For the two weeks that I couldn't drive, it was my only tie to the outside world. After that, I just needed it. I was still having many sleepless nights.

That afternoon, I was feeling pretty down so I called Geri to tell her how nervous and fearful I was about the discovery of the small amount of Stage III tissue. Most of the time, she had time to listen. I just had to talk about it, and I knew Bob had about had his fill, and I didn't want to burden him further. And right now, Katie, my best friend, was working.

Geri came to see me on Thursday. We had a nice chat, but she realized just the amount of anxiety I'm under and suggested a book that may help me. She tells me it's at some religious store, but I'm still feeling too weak to wonder and follow directions. My sense of direction had never been good. So, I ask her if she could pick it up for me and I would pay her back. The name of the book was *Getting Well Again* by the Simontons. Geri agrees to get the book for me. While we talk, she also notices that I'm down, which was not all that unusual under the circumstances, but I tell her that I'm disappointed that the people at work who had promised to come visit me while I couldn't drive hadn't shown up in the previous week. I was especially disappointed that Dani, another RN who I'd helped orientate and who I thought had become fairly close to me, hadn't come. She listened and empathized with my troubles. I offered her refreshment, but she declined which was probably a good thing since I didn't have any herbal teas or such.

The next day, Geri called and asked if she could come by about eleven as she had already bought the book that morning. I said, "Sure, but I have to pick up Ken. If I'm not there at exactly eleven, just wait a few minutes, because I should be back there shortly after."

I found Geri just sitting on the rock by a little pinon tree. Our yard was landscaped in Southwestern style with rocks encircling a small patch of grass. On the south end of the yard close to the little patio were some railroad ties and some big rocks surrounded by small stones around the pinon tree. It was a good place to sit if you had to wait. When I saw her, I asked if she had been waiting long. She said that she hadn't; that she had just sat down. I didn't see a car in the driveway or in front of the house, so I asked her if she had walked. She said that she hadn't; that her car was across the street. I asked her to come in. She came in for a little while but didn't stay long, as she had another commitment. She advised me to read the book. "It'll help you a lot," she said. I told her I could hardly wait to get started.

Ken bounced in the door dropping all his kindergarten paraphernalia on the floor as most little boys do and ran quickly out the door again screaming and yelling as he did this. I was glad my life was beginning to get back to normal but as I was still prone to headaches because of the residual tumor, I dreaded his coming home especially when he was extra noisy. Talking to the other kindergarten mothers who also picked up their children there was an activity I had resumed that I enjoyed. Karen loved to pick up Ken. She would run to him and give him a big hug. I always enjoyed seeing that.

I told Ken to please let Mommy rest a little while, and then I would get lunch. It was Karen who was hungry and kept persisting that I get lunch right away. I managed to rest for ten minutes or so before her requests turned to tears. While I lay across the bedspread in our room, I began to feel a little guilty. I had really dumped on Geri. I had told her that if it wasn't enough to have a brain tumor, the flu, and friends who didn't visit, I had also developed vaginal itching this week. She said, "You've really been through everything, haven't you? I guess when it rains, it pours." Then I thought, "Well she must have understood because she got the book for me, and she hugged me and wished me well when she left."

But just as I was feeling all down and out and lonely for a friend, who do you think called but Melanie? She always seemed to be around when I needed her. She called me once or twice a week since my surgery. I told her all the new problems I had encountered.

With feeling she said, "Oh, dear, I'm sorry, and you were doing so well." I complained that none of my work friends had come to visit me during the two weeks that I couldn't drive, that I had at least expected Dani as we had become friends when we worked there. She explained that they had been very busy, and maybe they were just a little tired. I said that it really didn't matter. What I really needed was another adult to talk to. I did talk to Bob once in a while, but he had taken over the laundry, cooking, and some of the housework, so he was often too tired to talk and would just escape into the TV and fall asleep.

On January 27th, I received a long-distance call from La Crosse, Wisconsin. The caller asked for Robert Cowden. I informed him that Bob wasn't home. Then he said, "I'm Curtis Brown, Director of Pharmacy at La Crosse's Lutheran Hospital. Would you tell Bob I've got a job opening working nights?" I told him that I would.

Bob and I had discussed moving to Wisconsin, so he and the children could be closer to his folks for a while. He had gone up to Madison last year to take his boards. I wasn't so willing to just pull up stakes and go, since we had put a lot into our house on Wellesley. So, I said, "If I agree to go, will you have a kitchen remodeled to my tastes?" He agreed. So, I persisted. "Will you get me a new car, silver with red trim?" He agreed. I still wasn't sure I was ready for the cold Wisconsin weather. So, I added, "How about a waterbed and a snowsuit?"

"Okay."

But, I continued, "If my arthritis gets real bad, or if Karen's health is threatened by her asthma, we'll have to move back right away." He said, "Of course. I love you."

I wasn't being greedy or trying to make it impossible for him to move. I just had to find out how sincere and committed he was to his wish.

When Bob came home, I told him the news. I had thought he would refuse because of the night shift, but to my surprise, he was excited and said if they offered him at least $23,000; he'd take the job. Bob called Curtis back, was promised the appropriate salary, and was told to report for work on March 5th.

My family had to find out about our move sooner or later, so I told my mom the next day and let her break the news to Dad, as I knew he would take it badly, thinking that Bob would be so cruel as to take me away so soon after my surgery. The person I didn't expect to take it all that badly was my sister, Carol.

Bob kept close communication with my doctor since they were all at Lovelace, where Bob worked. Dr. Golden wasn't a bit shocked about our upcoming move. He told Bob that as far as he was concerned, it was all right for me to travel. He had been a professor at Gundersen and would be able to recommend a good neurosurgeon. So, I had to let him know if I was going along with the family.

I had received many cards and letters from well-wishers the first week I was home from the hospital. Among them was a card from the kindergarten mothers, offering get-well wishes as well as their prayers, and a note from my sister Carol offering to do anything that would help me while I was convalescing. I also received an invitation from Mrs. Black, the kindergarten room mother, inviting all the kindergarten mothers for a tea without the children, a sort of reprieve from all the noise and frustrations that comes with being a parent. There was an RSVP number on the card.

I called Mrs. Black and informed her that I'd sure like to go but was not allowed to drive yet. She said she would contact one of the other mothers who lived by my area to pick me up.

It seems it was a bad year for kindergarten mothers. One of the mothers had a tumor on her kidney, which had to be surgically removed; another had a vaginal tumor, which also had to be removed. With so much tragedy among the kindergarten mothers, I think Mrs. Black wanted to extend some warmth among us and also give us a chance to get to know one another better. She also said she was relieved to know that my prognosis was good. She said that the other two ladies were doing well too.

January 31st turned out to be a perfect day for a party. It was bright and sunny, although the temperature was still cool, as it was only January. At about 9 o'clock in the morning, the mother who was to pick me up arrived in a brown and white blazer. I was still recuperating and felt nauseous, so I informed her that we might have to stop along the way. I had taken my Compazine (an anti-nausea drug) as I often had during the past few days, but my stomach was still queasy this morning.

The gal driving the blazer was a pretty but corpulent woman, her blond hair fixed up on her head with tiny wisps of curls on the side. Despite her size, she looked elegant. Pam introduced herself as did I. We talked a little about my surgery, and she told me about the two other girls who'd had tumors also.

It was a long drive to Mrs. Black's house, and I wondered why she sent her children to Queen of Heaven School. Anyway, we had a lot of time for talking while we rode. We eventually got to the subject of our moving to Wisconsin. She said she had moved from New Jersey, and her daughter was three at the time of the move. She said her daughter had a most difficult time adjusting to the move. Pam said that, even though she tried to decorate the little girl's room like the one she had back home, the girl could not adjust. She said that the room was as close as she could get it with the exception of the curtains, which she could not match as she couldn't find the material in Albuquerque. Despite her efforts, the little girl would cry and not sleep at night and, when she did, she would wet the bed. The other girl was older and what she had missed most was her friends. The baby boy, of course, didn't care except that his mother had to quit nursing him to cope with the other two. However, all babies are weaned at one time or another, so the move didn't affect him at all. She said the three-year-old had the hardest time. She advised me to let them get involved in the packing.

I told her I had given the kids each a box so they could pack what they really wanted to take. This was more of a chore than if I'd done it myself, but I had heard that it takes some of the sting out of moving. The kids kept packing and unpacking whenever they wanted to play with something in the box. However, I had started packing some of the toys and games in one of Ken's drawers just so. So, when they unpacked that, I lost my temper. It was so hard to pack and move, care for the kids, and keep my cool, especially when I wasn't feeling good at times.

She said that she thought I was doing amazingly well, and I told her that it was good to get a few things off my chest as I was in virtual isolation the past week except for phone calls and the kids. It was good to talk to another adult. Thank God it was almost over.

I don't usually open up to strangers but the loneliness and the camaraderie of the kindergarten mothers, and the sheer need to talk to someone who's already been there, caused me to reveal my concerns about moving.

We continued talking about children and were soon at Mrs. Black's house. It was located in a nice area in the Northeast Heights. The red brick house with dark-shingle, pitched roof lay nestled between two big poplars. We parked across the street from the house as some of the guests were already there and had taken the close parking spaces. We walked up the sidewalk to the front door, which opened to a hallway, and on the left was a kitchen decorated with bright reds and greens. I was surprised to see Miss McNeil, a pretty blond-haired girl with whom Ken had become infatuated with and also did very well with because "blonds were his type of girl." She was also a very good kindergarten teacher, dividing up time frames of fifteen minutes of one type of activity since kindergarteners' attention spans are limited. She also had them learn about the world from their own experiences so they would retain more information. Mrs. Abeyta, the teacher's assistant was also there. She had become fond of Ken and gave him an army hat, which he often played with at school before we left for Wisconsin.

On a card table, Mrs. Black had arranged an array of fancy cookies and pastries. The golden sun shone through the kitchen windows. The kitchen led to a dining room decorated in yellows and greens. On the dining room table was a fancy punch bowl with fancy-cut glass plates with an indentation for a cup. In the middle of the table was a big and finely decorated cake.

Since I was still nauseous, the only thing I wanted for the time being was punch. As I went around the room, I was introduced to several of the other mothers. I began to feel worse, so I began to look for a bathroom. When I found one, I promptly vomited but began to feel better—good enough to eat.

I washed up a bit then came out. I looked around and filled my plate with the luscious treats. Miss McNeil was standing by the table. She said she was sorry to hear we'd be going to Wisconsin. "It's so-o-o cold out there," she said. She said that she had moved from a northern state to come out here where it was warm.

"Why would you want to go there? I can't stand the cold."

"Neither can I. Bob's folks are out there, and he wants to spend a few years there so they can enjoy the children while they are still young."

Then we began talking about Ken. She said she liked Ken because he was so funny-he'd start to say something and go off on a tangent. One of the things he did during playtime was put on an army hat and march and sing about the room.

We parted to talk to some of the other mothers and have some cake. I got a piece of cake and chatted with Mrs. Black while she cut the cake. I asked her why she was sending her kids to a school so far away. She said that there was a teacher at their parish school that nobody could stand. Her oldest child had trouble with her, and she'd rather pay the extra tuition at another school than have her child get the same teacher, and yet she wanted the children to have a Catholic education. Then, we went on and talked about our sons. I revealed some of Ken's antics and how hard it was to keep up with him, especially now that I was sick. She said that her son was the easy child; that she had more trouble with her girl. Everyone kept telling me how good I looked for only being two weeks post-op.

Mrs. Black excused herself and went about being a good hostess offering everyone coffee or punch. I sat down on the step with one of the other mothers. I was getting tired. The house had a sunken living room that separated it from the dining room creating a long step between them. Even though the house was fancy, the atmosphere was informal, and we had no reservations about sitting there.

Once again, we talked about kids. We had a party to get away, and it seems all we could do is talk about them. But it was good to share some of the similarities and differences and how other parents handled the same problems.

We continued to mingle and at about twelve, people began leaving. We also gathered our coats to leave, thanked the hostess and I sought out Miss McNeil to say a special goodbye to her and to thank her for the special interest she took in Ken. Many of the mothers wished me good luck on the trip.

Pam and I left. As we pulled into my driveway, I thanked her for being so kind as to take me to the party. She said it was no trouble and hoped I would have better luck with Karen than she had with her daughter in moving. She said she believed that three was the worst age for moving. In a little over a month, Karen would be three, but I decided not to worry, yet, as I still had to think about recovering.

A bright new Monday arrived again much too early for my taste, but Bob didn't have to go to work until ten, so he sent Ken off to school. When I got up, I still lingered over my toast and milk. I began eating breakfast as Dr. Smith suggested, but I was still so nauseous that I could only manage to eat toast and milk. So, I delayed taking the Tegretol until I summoned up the courage to swallow the pill.

Things were getting better though, and I wasn't nauseous every day as I had been before, so I guess my body was slowly adjusting to the medication. But not everything was "hunky-dory." I still had my vaginal itch, so I called Katie, my best friend and nurse practitioner, and explained the problem to her. I said, "And if the tumor, the reaction to the medications, and the flu aren't enough I've got to put up with this terrible vaginal itch that's driving me crazy."

She asked, "Did you have any antibiotics, lately?"

"I don't know. Let me ask Bob." Fortunately, Bob hadn't left for work yet and I asked him.

He said, "Yeah, you had Kefzol in surgery." But before I had a chance to tell Katie that, she said, "Wait a minute. With all that you've been through, a monilial infection is possible." (A monilial infection is a yeast infection that occurs when the natural flora of a mucous membrane is wiped out.) I still informed her that I had Kefzol in surgery.

Katie said I should meet her at noon at Planned Parenthood the next day. We could have lunch, and then she could examine me. She forgot to give me directions since Planned Parenthood had changed locations recently. I called her back the next day at Planned Parenthood to ask her for directions. I told the woman who answered that Katie had scheduled me for twelve. She said she had no one scheduled at twelve and that Katie was with a patient at the moment. I told her I'd call back.

Bob overheard the conversation and said, "She's probably doing this on her own time, and you probably got her in trouble." I began to worry that I had gotten Katie in trouble, but I called back about fifteen minutes later apologizing sincerely if I had gotten her in trouble. She said that I hadn't gotten her in trouble; that they just don't usually schedule people at noon because that's when they take their lunch break. I was relieved and explained that the reason I had called was that I didn't know how to get to the new Planned Parenthood building. She gave me directions, explaining to go up Menaul past Wyoming until I saw a red brick building and that would be it. I wrote the directions down.

Karen and I set about 11 a.m. (I'm notorious for getting lost.) Bob didn't have to work until 3 p.m. that day so he could watch Ken until I got back. He had a weird schedule that changed times every day. So, I hopped in the car with Karen, and we set off. I drove down Menaul, slowly looking on the right side of the street for the red brick building. I didn't see it and went right past it until I realized that I had gone too far. I turned around in a parking lot and drove back slowly, looking more carefully. I finally gave up and called Katie from a gas station. It turned out I was very close, in the same block in fact. The reason I hadn't found it was because instead of facing toward the street it faced west. So, I drove a little way and parked.

Karen and I dismounted and headed for the door, but it was locked. Fortunately, a few minutes later, Katie saw us and unlocked the door. She said they closed from twelve to one and if they didn't lock the door, they wouldn't have any peace at that time.

There was a Spanish lady sitting at the desk that Katie introduced as Alvita. Katie left her keys with her, and we left the building to go have lunch. We were both harmonious and indifferent about our indecision, each hoping the other would make the decision. We finally settled on Annie's Soup Kitchen. We settled down on a molded yellow and green plastic booth. It had a refreshing atmosphere. Katie and I both had salads with crisp green lettuce with lots of helpings of red onions, mushrooms, tomato, garbanzo beans, green peppers, and carrots topped with Crispins and white turkey meat and cheese. Katie had hers with blue cheese dressing and I had mine plain as I never cared much for dressings and thought they covered up rather than enhanced the flavor of the vegetables. I just let Karen get what she wanted off my plate since it worked out cheaper that way since she doesn't eat much.

It was an enormous salad, and I was not able to finish it, even with Karen's help. I had asked for an extra plate this time. We left the restaurant and proceeded to the office. So, Katie and I left Karen playing while we went to the inner office. I chatted a stream of nervous chatter to hide my embarrassment. That was not like me. I'm usually quiet and reserved.

I had an uneasy feeling, not from the fear of the pelvic exam; I knew women practitioners were gentler, but the intimacy of the situation embarrassed me, since Katie and I were so close—so close that we perhaps should have been sisters barring that which may have destroyed the relationship.

Anyway, she showed me to a room, the typical OB-GYN exam room with the half-table with stirrups, a table with drawers that had instruments in front of the table, a window on one side, and a door on the other. She told me to strip to the waist, gave me a sheet, and said she'd be back in a few minutes. When she returned, I continued the conversation, which was about my recent operation. I seemed to have a need to mull it over many times in my mind, and many times just talking about it just to really believe that it had happened and start to get over it. It also relieved the slight and perhaps mutual tension in this situation.

I told her that Dr. Golden had offered me an injection of Ativan in order that I might forget most of the twenty-four hours surrounding the surgery. I had told him that I did want it. I told Katie that, although I had insisted on no drugs with the birth of my children, this was different and I didn't think I could handle it without the drugs. I also didn't care to remember the exact details. The painful memories that I had remembered were enough.

I don't know if it was all the nervous talk or just the fact that I was able to confide in Katie, but I discussed intimacies I would not have ordinarily discussed.

Katie made a slide and went to look at it under the microscope. She said she really didn't see an active monilial infection but just traces as if one was clearing up. She told me I could try Monistat Seven if I wanted. I told her I'd try it.

When we were done, I left the room and went to get Karen who was still playing with the toys in the corner and who would have stayed there all day if I let her. Toys other than their own always seem so much more fascinating to a child. I informed her that it was time to go.

She complained a little bit as Katie and I helped her put the toys back in the box. As we put on our sweaters to leave, I admired the macramé wall hanging. I told Katie that I had something like that in mind for her baby. Katie had confided in me that, now she had started in her nurse practitioner career, she was ready to have a baby. The heartwarming tidbit is that Katie and Dave decided to have children only after watching ours for a couple of years. When they got married, they had decided not to have children because the children they had known in the past were all brats.

The macramé wall hanging was three feet by two feet hanging with several rows of square knots expanding out into many rows of alternating square knots and then diminishing again into several rows of square knots. My idea was to take the example of the wall hanging and increase the size to three feet by three feet, attach a wooden frame leaving some slack for swinging purposes, and attach four macramé ropes which are tied to a ring for hanging. I thought that a baby swing would be a unique and ideal gift as I had already given them everything I had owned in baby equipment. But that idea would have to wait a while as I had to think about recovering and moving.

Karen and I had put on our sweaters. It was an early spring.

We told Katie, "Goodbye."

And she said, "Adios." The clinic was just beginning to stir as patients came in. We left.

Bob got the Monistat Seven for me the next day. I began to use it. The medication insert said that if the itching did not stop or increased in two days to discontinue the medication. I was so anxious for relief that I used it for three days. By the third day, [the] itching had intensified and the vanishing rash on my body reappeared. I thought (again) that I was allergic to the Tegretol. That medication had made me so miserable that I was willing to attribute any cause to discontinue it. What I hadn't realized until Bob pointed it out, [was] that the Monistat Seven could cause a systemic reaction by being absorbed through the mucous membranes.

I finally discarded the medication, called Katie to let her know what had happened, and let nature take its course. I was uncomfortable for a few more days, then began to feel better. Since it wasn't clear that I had a monilial infection, we both agreed that I should not take any more medication.

CHAPTER 5

I began to get cabin fever the second week post-op, when I was feeling better but still could not drive. I had few visitors that week, so I used the phone profusely when I did not sleep. After that, people began to come and visit me. Cards and flowers began to pour in. Our first and continually loyal visitors were Mom and Dad, and Katie and Dave, but mostly Katie.

I loved Katie to come because if I fell asleep, she was not the least bit offended. Mom and Dad came about every other day and later about twice a week. I appreciated Mom staying with me the first week, and I appreciated their concern. But after the first week, I became irritated with their visits for two reasons: (1) I wanted to start living a normal family life again, and (2) I was still quite sick and felt that they wanted to converse or be entertained, and I was still not feeling up to it. So, for a couple of their visits, I just stayed in my room. I told Bob to tell them I was very tired and wanted to rest. The second time I did that, Bob became angry with me and scolded me by saying, "What am I supposed to tell your folks when you refuse to see them?" I felt ashamed and tried to be more reasonable after that, but still wished that he could understand how I felt, since at the time I wasn't able to express my feelings in words.

When I was again able to drive, people began to visit. In this society, driving contributes to one's sense of independence. However, there were people who cared. Mrs. Jammee (the mother of Bob's best friend) brought a very large pot of chicken rice soup, saying that chicken soup cures anything. She also brought a platter of cookies and pastries for the children. She said that I could keep the yellow platter as she did not want it. I liked the chicken rice soup so much that later I asked her for the recipe. She brought it on a little card when she picked up her pot. I told Mom how much I liked the chicken soup that she had to bring me some too. By the time I finished what seemed like two gallons of chicken soup, I was ready to give it up for a long time.

Among all the well-wishers was my sister Carol, who had sent me a card saying, "If there's anything I can do for you, just let me know." I had become suspicious of Carol's new attitude since we had fought all during our growing years. But for the time being, I accepted her concern graciously and told her that I would call if there should be anything I need from her.

On January 30th, I received a call from Dr. Golden, personally. To say the least, I was surprised. Important doctors just do not call patients themselves; they delegate that responsibility to their secretaries. I suppose he called himself to keep what he was about to tell me confidential. He informed me that he had received a letter from my sister wanting to know just what was going on here. The letter said that she wanted to know the real condition of her sister. Dr. Golden had told her that a patient's medical record is confidential and that he could not give out that information without permission. He wanted to ask if I wanted him to give out the information or whether he should refer her to Bob, and if she had any questions. We opted for the latter choice, still unsure of what she was doing writing to my doctors. I wondered whether I could trust her.

On Monday, February 2nd, I had another appointment with Dr. Golden. The first thing he did was hold the letter up in the air, asking us if we wished to reconsider. Still unsure of Carol's purposes, we stood firm in our decision.

Dr. Golden then asked me how things were going. I said much better. He said, "Well, good. Then I'll call Dr. Roma (oncologist) and have you see him now as he is here today." He picked up the phone and called Dr. Roma, referring me to him. He then gave us directions to his office. It was a short visit.

As we strolled to Dr. Roma's office, I shared my suspicious feelings with Bob saying, "What do you think she's up to? She's never shown such concern over family?"

"I don't know. We'll just have to ask her, I guess. Knowing Carol, she has some ulterior motive."

Dr. Roma was waiting for us when we got to his office. He got out of his chair and met us at the doorway as we walked in. Dr. Roma was from Brazil. He is a rotund, short man with a black and grey mustache and beard. If his beard had been white, he would have looked like Santa Claus. He was a very warm and affectionate person, who put his arms around me and hugged me as he greeted us. Latin Americans are like that. They are brought up to be much more affectionate and open in their responses.

Dr. Roma made me feel warm inside and at home in his office. Just as he seated me in his office, he pulled Bob aside asking him how I took the news of a small amount of Stage III astrocytoma. Bob told him really well; that I was excited to start his program.

When he heard that, he told Bob to have a seat and started explaining about his program. Dr. Roma was a very relaxed man, swinging from side to side in his plush swivel chair with wheels. While he was talking to us seriously, he leaned forward, one hand clutched in the other, saying, "I guess you've been told that they reviewed your specimen again, and this time they did find..." I nodded my head. "Dr. Golden would like to have you try our pi meson treatment at Los Alamos. How do you feel about it?"

"Well, we've decided I should have the best treatment possible, and Dr. Golden and Melanie have told me that it is very pleasant there."

"Ahh, yes and we've had very delightful results. The only trouble is we don't know how successful it is on a long-term basis, since many patients come from all over the nation, they go all over, and we don't get a chance to follow them up for say ten years. And the people are very nice. You'll like it there," he drawled in a Latino accent.

He went on discussing the program and what I should expect,

saying that I might be awakened in the night when the machine was working, and that is why clients were to be available at all times. As he went on talking about the accommodations, he leaned back on his swivel chair, folded his hands, [and] stretched out his legs, crossing them at the ankles. He was so composed and at ease with himself and yet had a genuine concern for his fellow human being. I was so impressed with him that I spent most of the interview just watching him that I don't remember much of what he said except that I was to call Tami at the protocol office to set up an appointment with Dr. Schorr (radiation oncologist). He gave me a little card with the Cancer Treatment and Research Center number with Tami's name on it so I would know with whom to speak. All the while I was watching this man, I was subconsciously wondering how anyone could be so calm. He seemed to love everyone.

That week, my dad also surprised me and dropped in one morning. (He usually came in the evening with Mom, but now he was retired and had some free mornings.) He was alone and had brought me a pair of gloves saying it was a delayed Christmas present as he had been so busy fixing up the house that he couldn't get them over before. Actually, I believe it was his way of saying, "I love you; I'm going to miss you and I hope you don't freeze to death in that climate." Mom usually bought all the Christmas presents.

He had taken the news of our planned move to Wisconsin hard. He and Carol had reacted to the dreadful-sounding diagnosis and thought Bob was being cruel and inconsiderate. Actually, Bob and I knew I was in better health than they realized. Dad also knew he was losing his "little girl," even though he still had one at home. However, he always seemed to have great difficulty dealing with teenagers, and he and Joanie were going through that stage.[20]

After I got married and left home, though, he was much more affectionate. Still, I appreciated his concern for my health but felt that he was much more concerned over his distress over not seeing me as often as he would like over the coming years, which probably explains why my folks were over so much, in addition to my recent brain surgery.

---

20 Joanie is the name used to refer to Sandra's youngest sister.

When Dad wasn't over, he would sometimes phone. He would say, "I just wanted to be sure that you're alright. Sandra, are you sure you should move out there so soon after your surgery?" I'm sure he was thinking, "What if something would happen to you after you move?" I responded, with a little annoyance in my voice as he was asserting parental authority that he didn't have.

"Dad, we discussed our move with Dr. Golden. He isn't the least bit concerned. He's just glad that we're moving to an area where he can recommend a good neurosurgeon. Gundersen clinic is in La Crosse, which is a clinic with a pretty good reputation."

I felt the reason he made the telephone calls, instead of just expressing his opinion while he was visiting, was that he did not want Bob to consider him a meddler and did not want to actually accuse Bob of being cruel and inhuman.

My mother's attitude towards our move was much more reasonable. She told me while we were packing, "I won't object to your moving or try to get you to stay here. When your Dad was out of work and I was pregnant with you and couldn't work, we thought about going to California for your Dad to look for work. The opportunities were greater there. His dad talked him into staying, and I've always kind of regretted that."

On Wednesday evening, Bob came home and informed me that Dr. Golden had told him that my sister Carol had called him again requesting the information but that [Dr. Golden] had told her to ask us for any information that she wanted. I told Bob that was fine, but that I was becoming angry at her going to my doctors without even consulting me.

"Why couldn't she accept our word as the truth?" So, I called her, scolding her by saying, "What business is it of yours to call my doctors to request information? You can ask us. We're not hiding anything." She said that the pathologist at the hospital where she worked said that you had to be in danger of dying to be considered for the Los Alamos treatment facility. That cooled me down a bit as I started to understand where she was coming from. I didn't fully understand until we moved to La Crosse. So, I explained that I only had a small amount of Stage III tumor, perhaps only a cell or two as Dr. Golden had said. It's just that I'm a nurse working at the same facility that they are and feel a sort of kinship among us and would like to give me the best chance possible. Dr. Roma would even like to see how a patient with minimal Stage III responds to the pi meson. So, they left the choice up to me.

That seemed to satisfy her, and we were able to start over. I had begun to think of how I would go to Wisconsin after the treatments were over. I couldn't drive 1400 miles alone. So, remembering Carol's offer to do anything she could for me, I asked her if she would help me drive to Wisconsin when I had to leave.

Even though I had made my peace with Carol, I still had an uneasy feeling, perhaps not so much from her, as from my own fear of the unknown. That night, I again sat in the bean bag with Bob shaking with fear, telling him, "You won't let anyone take the kids away from me, would you?"

"Of course not. What made you say that?"

"Well, when I was talking to Carol earlier, she said she was very worried about my going to Wisconsin so soon after my surgery. She even said that you probably even took advantage of my illness and sold the house behind my back just so you could move to Wisconsin. I got angry and explained to her that the house was not sold; it was just put up for sale by a realtor and you could not sell the house without my knowledge, as I had to sign the papers to sell the house. I reassured her that we'd discussed the move with Dr. Golden, and he had no qualms about it. He was just glad we were moving to an area where he could give a good recommendation. She kept saying, despite my explanation, 'Are you sure you should move out there so soon after your surgery?' I told her that by the time I move there, it would be thirteen weeks after surgery. And I asked her to help me drive back to Wisconsin when I was through with the treatments since she said she would do anything for me. She said she had to talk it over with her husband Ben, and then she would let me know. She seemed sincere enough. Yet, I don't know. I kind of get an eerie feeling when she accuses you of selling the house. I think she might want something else, and I don't have money. The most valuable thing I have (other than you) is the kids.

Maybe she'd try to declare me incompetent and take them."

"Don't worry. She can't do that without my help." He then hugged me and kissed me for a while. After a few minutes, I began to feel better and went to bed. While in bed I began to ponder why Carol showed this over-concern. What came to mind was not the thoughts I had discussed with Bob before, but maybe she was moving back to Albuquerque the next year and she would miss the opportunity to see me more often, especially if the pathologist in Kansas City had given her the impression that I would die if I didn't get the treatment, or in spite of it.

Whenever I had any problems like this, I called Katie, but it was so late, I planned to call her the next day. Katie, a true friend, was always willing to listen and often had an encouraging word. I called Katie the next day. "Can you imagine calling someone else's doctor and demanding confidential information?" I exploded.

"We're talking about Carol, I assume."

"Yes, remember I told you that she had written a letter to Dr. Golden in order to find out what my 'real' condition was."

"Uh-huh."

"Well, that wasn't enough for her. She had to go and call him too. She didn't learn anything new. We told Dr. Golden to tell her to ask us if she had any questions. She even thought Bob sold the house while I was ill. Now isn't that dumb to think that he could sell the house without my even knowing about it? I told her that he couldn't do that because I had to sign the papers to sell the house, too. Why do you think she'd do all this?"

"Well, you know she's so far away and wants to do something but feels helpless to do anything, so she probably called the doctor in desperation."

"Ya, but you'd think with her brains she'd know that medical information is confidential and that you can't sell a house without both partners consenting."

"Well, she's going to miss you. She was probably looking forward to seeing you next year, and now she's disappointed that you'll be even further away, and she doesn't want you to move. I don't want you to move either, but I know you have to do what you have to do."

"I'm going to miss you so much, too."

"I'll write, promise."

"I don't know. It just seems that she is so unduly concerned. Of course, I'm very concerned also, but she seems worse. When I asked her to help me drive to Wisconsin, she said she was concerned about complications. She acts as if I'm going to have an aneurysm."

"Well, it could happen…"

"Well, it's not going to. Did I tell you Geri came by and brought me the book Getting Well Again? It's about how to cure illnesses through meditation. It mostly talks about cancer, but states that you can cure other illnesses too."

"I know of one lady who cured her own brain tumor by saying each day that a little bit of her tumor was gone each day. She eventually cured herself."

"That's great. It's nice to know that someone you knew actually did it." We bid each other goodbye until we saw each other again. Sometimes we were on the phone for over an hour, but I never thought the time was wasted.

The rest of the day, I spent packing what I could and just feeding and playing with the kids. I never tackled any big packing job while I was alone. That evening, Sally and another neighbor lady whom I hadn't met yet dropped in unexpectedly. She had gotten together with the neighbors to get me a get-well card and a beautiful white gown with an empire-style bodice trimmed in blue-grey lace at the bodice and hem. It was a very elegant nightgown, I thought. How thoughtful of them to think of me in a time like this.

I invited them to come in. They came through the door, stayed long enough to see me open the present, then quickly excused themselves saying they didn't want to tire me. I thanked them and told them how thoughtful it was to think of me and to thank the other neighbors too.

I also got cards in the mail. One of them was from the kindergarten mothers again offering to do whatever possible to help. They also offered their prayers that I should make a complete recovery. The old saying of "in time of need, a friend indeed" was true of these ladies. They even asked Bob at the church parking lot where we picked up Ken if they could cook or babysit. Bob told him that he was a pretty good cook, and that Sally was always there when we needed a babysitter, but that he appreciated the kindness anyway. He got so many offers to bring food that he thought people thought he couldn't cook.

Mom and Dad Cowden were also very concerned, and they sent a card as well as a nice flannel orange gown. It seemed everyone thought that I was going to spend a lot of time in bed. When I was in the hospital, Katie's mother brought a bed jacket, which although I appreciated the concern, I returned to Katie as soon as I could drive, telling her that I wouldn't be needing it anymore. The unintentional hints to classify me as an invalid just intensified the flames of [my] desire to get well quickly. After the Tegretol level dropped to a reasonable level, I no longer stayed in bed, except to perhaps read *Getting Well Again*, as I wanted to finish the book and start on the program.

I was still in bed on Friday, February 6th, when I got a call from Alexander Jack. I was not sleeping but was just taking my time in getting up as I was still reading my book. Once I really got started, I had a hard time stopping. I knew I had to do it. When Mr. Jack first said who he was, I was a bit confused as to why he would want to call me. But he explained that he and Willie, his wife, had been praying for me and that he was the minister of his church, and that he often called people in time of need, to be there when they needed them. It was then that I first mentioned writing about my experiences. At the time, I was thinking of a *Readers Digest*-type article, but he encouraged me to write down my experiences and feelings day by day on 3x5 cards and then when it came to actually writing, it would be so much easier. I did admit that I had been through a lot but was not yet ready to open up and express my feelings to him, as I felt I did not know him well enough yet.

But I did need a support group as the time grew nearer to when Bob would leave for Wisconsin, and I would go to Los Alamos. One of my confidantes was Alice, another friend who was easy to talk to as we had shared the "trials and tribulations" of raising kids of the same ages. I had called her also because she was an "up" person, who could always see the brighter side of the coin.

On this particular occasion, I called her and told her I had reservations about going to Los Alamos; I feared that being surrounded by people who all shared the same misery would depress me. I wondered whether they talked of their illness all the time and whether I could cope in such an environment at a time when I would have no family or friends to comfort me. I didn't know if I could stand the loneliness. I told her that I did look forward to coming home on weekends and visiting Mom and Dad and Joanie and Katie.

She came up with a very reasonable explanation. She said, "Nah, there must be some 'up' people there who could befriend you. And who'd want to talk about their disease all the time anyway?" That made sense. I would have to avoid the people who would depress me and socialize with the 'up' people.

I also told her that I was nervous about going to the Cancer Treatment and Research Center; that both Melanie and Dr. Golden had said that would be the hardest part of all. They would treat me like a cancer patient.

That night, I told Bob that I was not looking forward to going to the Cancer Treatment Center. I also expressed the feeling that it was sure going to be lonely without them. He often joked about my going to Los Alamos saying, "You'll probably pick up some guy, while I'm out there working."

To which I would respond, "<u>Sure</u>, I'd just <u>love</u> to pick up some guy who's probably going to die, right?" Then, he would continue saying that I didn't have to pick up a patient, I could go after a doctor or a psychologist.

"Right," I would respond sarcastically. But seriously, I plodded, "Besides being lonely, I was wondering how Karen will take a seven-week period without me. She's only two you know. I'm also worried about getting sick. (A common side effect of radiation therapy is nausea and vomiting.)

"I've been thinking about that too. What I was thinking is why don't you keep Karen down there with you? She wouldn't miss you and you wouldn't have time to think about getting sick; you would have to stay well in order to take care of her."

"I like that idea. Do you really think they'll let me keep her?"

"I don't know why not. A relative can stay, can't they? Just tell them that you intend to keep Karen when you go down there."

He lifted my chin and asked seriously this time, "What am I going to do without you for seven weeks?" His jokes, I feel, were his way of dealing with the anxieties and frustrations of living without me for a while.

"There's still the problem of where I'll be staying for two weeks. Tami, Dr. Schorr's secretary, said the next group begins therapy on March 9th. I was thinking of asking Katie if I could stay with them for two weeks."

"Sure, or I'm sure your Mom and Dad, or Jane and my brother, or even John Schilling. He offered to let you stay there."[21]

"I'd feel more at home with Katie, I think. Even at Mom's, there'd be a strain, I think. It would be fun to stay with my brother, though. I could help with the babies since I won't be working. Still, I think I should ask Katie."

Monday, February 5th was my appointment at the Cancer Research and Treatment Center. The dreaded day had come. Though I dreaded going there, I dragged myself over to the center. I had already experienced how depressing a place it was since I had once accompanied a patient there.

My appointment was for 10:30 but I was informed by the receptionist to be there at least by 10 since I was a new patient and she needed to get extra information and make out a CRCT card. I also had a one o'clock appointment with Dr. Schorr.

I arrived promptly at 10 as requested. It never pays to be early. What do you suppose happened? Did they rush me through since I had arrived early in order to speed up the process? No, first I had to wait in line for fifteen minutes while a receptionist talked to another patient. Then, when she finally got to me, she sent me to another woman in the next stall who was talking on the telephone,

---

[21] It is not clear who Jane, my brother, and John Schilling are in this paragraph. Sandra changed the names of family and friends, and these names are not identifiable.

so I waited another fifteen minutes while she gabbed. Finally, she got off the phone, but by then it was 10:30, the time I was to have arrived in the first place. But I let my impatience go unnoticed, as it probably wasn't her fault. Then, after getting my name, address, phone number, and insurance number, etc. (I gave her Katie's phone and address and Mom's phone number and listed them both to notify in case of an emergency.) she started discussing finances, which I was totally unprepared for.

I told her, "I thought the treatment was subsidized by the government."

"True," she said, "but that covers only the treatment and your room. Any other service is your responsibility to pay."

"What other services are you talking about?" I inquired.

Then, another woman who'd overheard the conversation and the woman who was interviewing me said simultaneously, "The doctor's exam here and any other test or service performed at this facility."

"And it doesn't include any tests they may run or any medication you may need." I signed the form she gave me indicating that Bob and I would be responsible for any extra bills. I handed her my Blue Cross/Blue Shield Insurance card.

She went on to say that she wanted to make it clear that the insurance might not cover all outpatient charges. I informed her that I was aware of that, but I wanted to submit the insurance for any charges that they could cover.

"Of course," she said. She also made out an ID card for CRTC which she said I was to present any time I came there and that it allowed me to park in the reserved area in front of the center for cancer patients. I told her that I hoped this would be the last time I had to deal with them since my treatment was to take place in Los Alamos.

She then sent me to Tami whom Dr. Roma said I would see. She was in charge of coordinating the Los Alamos facility with CRCT. When I arrived at her office, I met another girl who shared the office. When I asked for Tami, she informed me that Tami was on her lunch break.

"Have a seat. She'll be back in a few minutes." I waited another 15 minutes, which seemed like an eternity. While I was waiting, I decided to occupy myself by reading the posters they'd hung on their bulletin boards and the pictures they had on their desks. I was angry over all the inefficient service they had given me, and I was also getting hungry as lunchtime grew near. But, I sat in silence reading the posters as this girl was not responsible for their inefficiency. The posters were humorous but did not seem so as they poked fun at the way the operation was run, like, "Don't ask me, I only work here."

However, I was polite to the girl in the office and made small talk about the babies in the pictures. She told me a little about her baby and asked if I had any kids. I replied, "A boy who is five and a girl of two."

She said, "You're lucky to have a boy and a girl. With my luck, I'll get another boy." She terminated the conversation on that note and went on about her work.

As I continued reading the messages on the posters, Tami abruptly walked in. She startled me when she said, "Hello!" Then, noticing the slight jump, apologized, saying, "Oh, I didn't mean to scare you."

"It's okay," I replied. "I've been a little jumpy, lately."

She called Dr. Schorr to tell him I was there. Then she began to tell me about the living arrangements. I would have a room with a small kitchenette where I could cook. She said the room was subsidized by the government, but I was to buy my own food. She asked me a few questions; the same ones that were asked at the receptionist's office. I was getting tired of answering the same questions over and over. Then she handed me some forms to fill out. One of them was a psychological questionnaire. I told her that I had been talking to Melanie Brooks and that we had a good rapport, and I hoped this form wouldn't mean that I had to talk to someone else. I also feared exposing my private life so openly, as I didn't know who might read this. But I didn't tell her that. She responded that Melanie had worked for them and had been in on making the form. I was still reluctant to fill it out. She said it was just a survey for a research study. Reluctantly, I filled it out.

She gave me directions to Dr. Schorr's office. When I got there, there seemed to be no one around. Finally, I saw a woman and told her I was there to see Dr. Schorr. She asked me my name.

When I told her, she said, "I think you belong in here (pointing to an examining room) but let me check. Two other ladies walked up the hallway about that time. She said, "Wait here a minute." And then went to talk to them. When she came back, she said, "Yes, we want you in here." Then she told me to remove all of my clothing except my panties and gave me a white gown to put on.

I said, "It's awfully cold in here; is he going to be long?"

She said, "I don't know. He's an awfully busy man. You better put it on now before he comes." I did as I was told but was left with the feeling that he was the type of doctor who kept everyone waiting but would yell and holler should anyone keep him waiting. As I expected, it was a long wait. The longer I waited, the colder I got and the angrier I became.

When Dr. Schorr finally came in, he found me sitting, with my arms huddled around myself.

The first thing he said was, "You're cold?"

I nodded my head.

"It is rather chilly in here," he said without so much as a hint of emotion.

He was a cold young man, probably in his thirties, slim physique with blonde hair and a receding hairline, and stiff upper lip. He was wearing a white lab coat. He reminded me of an old-fashioned disciplinarian type of schoolteacher I've seen on TV. I could just imagine him walking around the room holding a ruler in one hand, slapping the other one as he gave a lecture.

As I glared at him, he received my vibes of a cold reception and said, "My name is Dr. Schorr. Is something wrong?"

"No, I've only been waiting forty-five minutes in this thin gown in this icebox," I said sarcastically.

He gave the typical reply that he was very busy and added that he had to see twenty patients the one day a week that he was in Albuquerque. Then he told me to get on the table.

Choking down the lump in my throat, I took a deep breath and did as I was told. I didn't say another word, as I was not going to let this man see me cry. And I didn't mention that I planned to keep Karen in Los Alamos with me. I could see that he had no heart.

He put his cold stethoscope under my left breast and listened to my heart, then he moved it around my chest listening to my breath sounds. He then proceeded to my back and told me to take several deep breaths. Again, I did as I was told. Satisfied that my heart and lungs were healthy, he began to ask me questions.

"This says you've been diagnosed as having a brain tumor, midline, astrocytoma Grade 2 and 3. Drs. Golden and Smith explained [the] meaning of this?" I nodded my head in the affirmative.

"Tell me what happened. Did you have headaches?"

"Yes, but I did not suspect anything serious as I treated them as sinus headaches and the treatment worked. Just as I had made an appointment to see a doctor, I switched antihistamines and started using a vaporizer. I described the headaches to Drs. Golden and Smith. They told me that they sounded like sinus headaches. I had no way of knowing."

"Go on…"

"Well, I was working. We had delivered a compromised infant; I went to lunch and the next thing I remember was waking up in the emergency room. And the emergency room doctor was telling me I had a seizure."

"Have you had any more?"

"No."

"Any headaches?"

"Of course, I've got kids."

"You had surgery a month ago?"

"Yes."

He proceeded in doing a neuro-check looking into my eyes for any evidence of neuro damage. Using a penlight, he continued the exam, darkening the room and watching the contraction of my pupils. Then he turned on the light and checked for peripheral vision by stretching his arms out, [and] wiggling his thumbs while instructing me to look straight ahead and asking me if I saw both thumbs.

"Do you have any vision problems?"
"No."
"Seeing double?" (I guess he didn't believe me.)
"No." Continuing his exam he put [up] different numbers of fingers several times. After the third try, after having given him the right answers, he gave up and proceeded to check my reflexes. He was very thorough in that.
"Of course," I replied. He seemed disappointed or puzzled that he hadn't found any symptoms to coincide with my chart.
In a monotone, he said, "I've found no neurological deficit, but you have a serious diagnosis, so I'd like to get you started as soon as possible. Our next protocol begins March 9th. "Who is going to be staying with you?"
"No one."
"Are you sure? You might need someone to stay with you. Can't your husband stay with you for at least the first week."
"No, we're moving to Wisconsin and he's leaving the 21st."
"Can't he postpone it for a week?"
"No, he starts work March 5th."
"Well, maybe you could get someone to stay with you. Think about it. And drop by Tami's office on the way out so she can get things started."
So, I got dressed and went back to Tami's office. While I slowly ambled down the long hallway (I wasn't about to hurry for these people), Dr. Schorr buzzed Tami on the intercom as I left to notify her of my arrival.
When I returned to her office, she said, "You'll be starting with the March 9th group, but we'll have to schedule you for a CAT scan before that." She called someone a couple of times to see if the helicopter was available. Apparently, it wasn't as she told me, that she would call me when the helicopter was ready and when she had scheduled the CAT scan. She also said, "We can fly you free or you can have someone drive you as you'll probably be drowsy, afterward."
"I'll fly."
She went on to explain the living arrangements. She said that the

government provided a small apartment for one or two people. She asked who was going to stay with me. I told her I intended to keep Karen, my daughter, with me.

"You can't do that! It's against the rules," she said excitedly.

"But she's only two. Just think of the emotional turmoil a separation of seven weeks would cause."

"With your diagnosis, anything could happen. What if you should have to go to the hospital? What would you do with her? Besides, our insurance would not cover her for anything that could happen."

"Isn't there anything you can do to let her stay with me?"

"I'll call Dr. Schorr, but I doubt it."

She pressed the intercom button on the telephone, which was busy. So, after trying a few more times, she was connected with him. She said, "Mrs. Cowden wants to keep her daughter with her in Los Alamos. I told her that we couldn't because it was an insurance risk. But she's very worried about being away from her 2-year-old for seven weeks." There was silence while he talked. She hung up the phone and said, "Just as I thought. We can't do it because of the insurance risk."

"I've been taking care of her for the last two weeks and nothing's happened to her," I choked out. "I'm going to ask Dr. Smith if there's anything that can be done." As I spoke, my heart sank. I just couldn't leave my baby for that long. I just hoped Dr. Smith could find a way out of this situation. I hoped it was not futile. I must have drifted off in my thoughts because she said, "Sandy?"

"Yes?"

"We'll let you know when we'll fly you to Los Alamos for the scan."

"Okay." Fuming inside, I left without saying goodbye. I was very resentful over losing control of my life. People who I didn't even know were making the important decisions in my life, even my appointments. They told me when to come, not asking whether it was convenient. To think that they wouldn't even let me have my own daughter with me was unthinkable, and at the very least, downright infuriating. I made up my mind that one way or another I wasn't going to let this happen. First, I was going to tell Bob, then

Melanie, and then Dr. Smith.

When I got home, Bob asked me how it had gone. I exploded, "They act as if I'm dying, and they said I couldn't keep Karen with me. She said, 'You can't keep her there with your diagnosis,' then she went on to say that it was against the rules and that they couldn't because it was an insurance risk."

Bob said, "Let me see what I can do. I mentioned it to Dr. Smith, and he thought it was a good idea. I'll talk to him in the morning."

I was not patient enough to wait until morning. I had a sense of urgency to do something, so I called Melanie and told her that they were not going to let me keep Karen with me.

"Why not?" she asked.

"Because they say it's against the rules..."

But Melanie, already furious, interrupted saying, "Rules are made to be broken. I'll see what I can do." I felt somewhat better, relieved to get things off my chest, and felt that I wasn't totally losing control over my life. I could at least pressure them to reconsider.

CHAPTER 6

On February 7th, a bright and cool day, Mom and Jane came over to help me pack. Bob had started packing and I helped whenever I felt like it, and that was not much. But the boxes were already out when Mom arrived early that afternoon. She said that we would start with things we would not need. So, we started with the china, which was in the china hutch easy enough for Mom to do without much help. She asked me where the towels were that I didn't need so she could wrap the dishes up in them. I went to the linen closet and brought a stack of towels saying, "I hope this is enough." I helped for about half an hour and then began to feel very drowsy, the kind of drowsy I could do nothing about. I told Mom I was just too tired to go on, lay on the couch with my comforter, and fell asleep. Mom made a quick lunch with the small amount of food and utensils that were left unpacked. Jane arrived at about one in the afternoon. She had a lot of good ideas as she had moved from Trinidad, Colorado to Albuquerque when she married my brother.

After Jane arrived, we began to pack the small appliances. We used linens to pack fine breakables. Jane had left her son with my brother. Bob was keeping Ken busy with various little jobs, and Karen was his assistant in helping sort out things in the garage as to what they wanted and what they didn't. So, we had a good time chatting and packing.

Jane had to leave at about four, but I thanked her sincerely.

"Without you two," I told Mom and Jane, "I would never have

done it." It was beginning to look like we would get all packed in time. Mom stayed until about suppertime. I thanked her again. I was glad we had accomplished so much, and though the workload ahead of us was still great, we had put a dent in it. I was slowly recovering. I was now helping Bob fix dinner and setting the table.

Sunday was a calm, quiet family day. I only packed a few things that morning, as I had told Bob I was only going to pack when I felt like it. He was very understanding and said that I didn't have to pack anything if I didn't want to, [and] that he'd get it done. I didn't want to be a malingerer or put all the burden of this move on his shoulders, so I packed when I had little bursts of energy. I rested when I was weary. I had put together a simple lunch. Bob and I had put a few dishes in the dishwasher and were relaxing in the living room near the warm glow of the fireplace hearth. Bob was in the bean bag chair in front of the TV, and I was in the lounge chair reading the Sunday paper. The doorbell rang. I expected Jack or one of the neighbor kids as we were always going back and forth. But it turned out to be my uncle and his wife. I was surprised. I had never expected them to come, and above all, I hadn't expected the feast they brought; turkey and dressing, mashed potatoes and gravy, a salad and cranberry sauce, and an apple pie all in disposable paper plates and dishes so we wouldn't have to return anything later. They stayed a few hours that afternoon to visit.

They had not been informed of our impending move when they arrived but were not dismayed or discouraged about our leave. In fact, they saw it as a fresh start for both of us. They said it would probably be easier to get over this crisis by being away from the family and being constantly reminded of it. For me, it was refreshing to hear a different point of view. I was in need of a positive attitude.

The rest of the afternoon, we just spent chatting and enjoying Karen's antics. She loved to show off in front of company. They left about four saying that they wanted us to enjoy that meal. We invited them to share it with us as it was too much for us. They insisted that they brought that for us, and they wanted us to have it, so we bid them goodbye and thanked them sincerely for their generosity.

We ate well that night, remarking on how this was like a

Thanksgiving dinner. They had brought the whole turkey, not just some slices.

Katie and Dave came over that evening, and I finally could carry on a decent conversation without falling asleep. Bob added wood to the fire. I was getting the kids ready for bed and although they usually tried to procrastinate, they cooperated whenever Katie and Dave were around. It seemed they always wanted to impress them. I told them to go and give "Aunt" Katie and "Uncle" Dave a night-night kiss. Karen had to have Dave, whom she called "Daddy" a bedtime story. She sat upon his lap with her book open in her sleeper, content as could be just listening to the story. I thought it was very sweet and heartwarming, just the two of them sitting on the recliner reading a story that I had to take a picture of them. Although I thought it was sweet for Karen to call Dave "Daddy," I took a lot of ribbing about it.

Bob teased me saying, "I've been meaning to talk to you about this."

I usually retorted back, "Your kids look just like you; you couldn't deny them if you wanted to." (The amazing thing was that Aunt Carol had picked Ken out of the many babies in the nursery without having seen his nametag first. We were standing at the nursery window, and she said, "That's him, that's Bob's baby.")

Monday came, and I continued packing as before. In his spare time, Bob was sorting out things in the garage. It's amazing how many things you can collect in seven years. Mom came over in the afternoon to help me pack. She had taken half a day off to do this. I told her I had to go over to the hospital to finish things off, so I asked her to come with me to resign and make arrangements for any disability pay that I might be eligible for having become ill on the job.

We went to the fourth floor to Kathy Browner's office (head nurse of pediatrics) where Jacquelyn, my head nurse happened to be at the time. I introduced my mom to them and started to ask whether or not I was eligible for any compensation for getting ill on the job.

Mom interrupted and said, "Workman's compensation."

Jacquelyn said, "Not workman's compensation, but temporary disability insurance." The hospital had already put in and received approval for thirteen weeks of disability insurance. She suggested I resign as of May 1981, so as to ensure getting all of the payments.

Katie came after work at about four o'clock. She was kind of apologetic for not being able to come and help on Saturday as I had asked. I assured her that she need not feel guilty; I did not expect her to pack for me but just appreciated any help I could get. We began taking pictures from the walls and some of the decorative pieces on the bookshelves and off the fireplace mantel. I began to feel nostalgic as the house began to empty, but never dreamed how much I would miss the fireplace.

All that week, we packed as I was getting stronger. Our home seemed to be like the changing seasons, once in full bloom of spring and summer-every picture, portrait, and knick-knack in just the right place. After moving in with only a card table for eating and two folding chairs to sit on, lawn furniture in the living room, and an old trailer bed we'd bought from Bob's cousin to sleep on, we'd finally made this our home, our castle. We had taken advantage of bargains and sales on furniture. It was not elegant, but it was us and it was attractive, our personalities fused and permeated our essence throughout the house. Bob surprised me one day by buying a Mediterranean bedroom set. I liked the heavy dark wood but had been a bit disappointed that I hadn't helped in choosing it, but I did not mention it at the time. He also got a bargain on some more Mediterranean dining room furniture, a large rectangular table with a leaf, six chairs, and a finely carved china hutch. Again, I was somewhat disappointed over not choosing the furniture, though I liked it. This time, however, it occurred to me that if I didn't mention that I would like to take part in furnishing the house, he would have furnished the whole house without my input. So, I told him I liked the furniture. The chairs had false caned backs, which I thought were attractive. So, we went together to buy a dinette set. I chose the kitchen table, which was a false marble blue Formica, hexagonal with plush overstuffed bright blue vinyl swivel chairs. I also chose our living room furniture: a couch, loveseat, and armchair with a modern-striped design with a sturdy oak frame which I thought was practical because we planned [to have] children and did not want something expensive. If it were to be ruined, we would not have wasted a lot of money. The whole set was under $300. Bob had also surprised me with a red velvet armchair that he knew I wanted. But it was not so much the big furniture that reflected our aura, it was the little things that we had each contributed to make our house a home. So, we began to take such things as the "neecie," a brass candlestick, and a collection of decorative candles, an old-fashioned flue for adding oxygen to a fire, and a brass Aladdin's lamp, which was finely decorated with carved flowers and leaves, surrounded by a delicate red and green design, and a glass donkey pulling a cart from the mantle of the fireplace. Beside the fireplace, I had a shelf that held a hand-painted Indian vase, with a black and orange American Indian geometric design, an old-fashioned oil lantern, one of our many photographs, and some grandma and grandpa dolls. Some of these items had been given to us, and some we had collected on one of our trips to Wisconsin. A "neecie" is an elf that legend says takes care of the house and sometimes does work for the owner. We took these treasures down, wrapped them in towels or newspaper, and put them in boxes, labeling the box with the room they came from. We also packed Bob's collection of mortars and pestles. Down came our own little contributions to the house such as the macramé plant hangers I had made, the wooden plaques to hold such antiques as a horseshoe, and a railroad nail that he had made for Ken. We had bought a light with a ceiling fan for the dining room because it looked good and because it redistributed the heat in the house, but that was staying. We also packed the Indian rugs I bought, again using them to pack more fragile items. Autumn had come; our little treasures were coming off of the wall and going into boxes on the floor, creating a maze that we had to tread when we wanted to go from one room to another.[22]

The rest of the week, I continued packing and had developed a routine of getting up with the children and fixing breakfast. I continued eating a light breakfast, dawdling over it as I was still

---

22 This is Sandra's metaphor about moving from New Mexico to Wisconsin (during February of 1981).

hesitant to take the Tegretol. I found that I like C.W. Post cereal dry, or two pieces of toast and a glass of milk seemed to settle my stomach the best. I had now come to believe that maybe I did need more nutrition to fight off the fatigue as well as the nausea.

I would get Ken out of the door after breakfast. I had him dressed before breakfast as he tended to meander around the house to the television, play make-believe games, or just run around the house wildly whooping and hollering. Sometimes disagreements over the morning routine escalated into fights as my fuse was still short, especially when I had a headache. (The headaches continued as they could not remove the entire tumor.) Ken was also a difficult enough-to-handle child when I was well. He was at least borderline hyperactive, and I hadn't yet learned to deal with it well.

After Sally had picked up Ken, I would either lay on the bed and read or sit in front of the TV with Karen watching Sesame Street. Sometimes, I would still fall asleep there. When I did, it gave me new energy to continue packing.

What I was learning from reading *Getting Well Again* was that I had participated in my illness. I became an avid reader wanting to know all about the "imagery process" which contributed to the cures of many patients. Yet, I had to maintain a household, pack, care for the children, and still recover from the Tegretol overdose. But I read whenever I had the chance. One half of me desperately wanted to believe that I could cure myself, but the other half still had doubts. The book had eventually become my security.

Another thing I was learning was that there was more than one factor in my life which permitted the tumor to start to grow, six to eighteen months before the disease became obvious. The book states that clusters of psychological stress in a person's life over which he feels he had little or no control over may lead to feelings of despair or depression which activate the "fight or flight" mechanism which causes changes in hormones that suppresses the body's immunological system so that cancer or atypical cells are not killed.[23] [Below is an important note on the etiology of cancer.]

I began to reflect upon my life eighteen months before January of 1981. Eighteen months previously was July 1979. [In] July of 1979, I was working at Bernalillo County Medical Center (now UNM hospital) on the postpartum unit. I was working the 3-11:30 shift. On average, we had eighteen or nineteen patients in our unit with at least four C-sections, two of them fresh with IVs and Foley catheters. (Sometimes they had more than these problems.) We had at least two high-risk ante-partum patients and always one or more newly delivered ladies who had to be transferred and sized, showered, vital signs taken upon transfer, and one hour later, and then settled in bed. We also usually kept the IV in for a while, just in case she bled. To do this amount of work, we usually had three people on duty—an RN, an LPN, and a nursing assistant. For a routine postpartum unit with no C-sections or high-risk antepartum, the staffing would have been fine. The workload was greatly increased by having these patients on the unit.

Patient care was not the only work involved. The doctors, residents, and med students arrived on scene at 4 p.m., changing orders and seeing patients at the time, often requesting information of the patients. We worked as rapidly and efficiently as we could under the circumstances, often having to choose what was to get done on the basis of priorities. (Example: A patient who was bleeding heavily had to be taken care of first.) So, on extremely busy evenings some of the household chores of picking up trash and filling ice pitchers were neglected. This was not often, and mistakes were occasionally made, as we are only human. But if anything was out of place or just not perfect, the night nurse would get irritated so much so that she had to run and "tattle" to the

---

23 It is worth noting that there is no scientific evidence that stress or depression leads to cancer or an inability of the immune system to kill cancer cells. Cancer is caused by mutations in DNA leading to uncontrolled cell growth. Dr. Simonton's book says that imagery and meditation can improve the healing process. As a cancer researcher I do not support the idea that cancer can be cured through meditation. However, meditation and counseling can be incredibly beneficial to cancer patients' emotional state. At the time this was written, it was not known that mutations in DNA are the cause of cancer.

head nurse. The head nurse realized how petty the night nurse could be. She, fortunately, sorted out the complaints before she said anything to the evening staff.

I might have been able to handle the stress caused by the heavy workload, but I could not handle the stress caused by the night nurse. She seemed to have some personal grievance against me. Most of the staff had trouble relating to her, but when she just glared at me, I felt the hatred cutting through me like a sharp knife. It also intimidated me so that I'd lose concentration on my report and make mistakes. The overall effect was that I wanted to get done with it as soon as possible.

Her piercing stare made me feel as though she wanted to kill me. It was not just her stare that caused so much stress. She seemed to be purposely trying to trip me up. She would often snap and make curt remarks.

At the head nurse's suggestion, we tried to reconcile our differences by talking them out. I told her I just could not give a good report when her attitude was so openly hostile. She said that she was not my mother and didn't have to cater to me. I informed her that I did not expect her to be my mother but would only like some professional courtesy during report. After a long, heated discussion, we agreed for her to be less threatening, and for me to double-check my information. Although we both improved slightly, still a hostile feeling left a coolness in the relationship. I was not happy at having to give her report, and I was unable to express the anger I felt toward her in front of her. Even in our discussion, I held back my emotions not letting her see just how angry I was, leaving me with a lump in my throat.

Suppressed anger is one of the factors the book states may precipitate cancer.[24] I had worked there a year and a half, and the combined stress of working in a very short-staffed unit, and the added stress of the night nurse's attitude had me so uptight that, by the end of the year, I was beginning to think about leaving the

---

[24] Anger does not mutate DNA or cause cancer. But at the time the causes of cancer were unknown, so I can understand why a book may incorrectly speculate that stress and anger contribute to cancer.

place. I had heard through the grapevine that she would make sure I could not transfer anywhere else in the hospital. I don't know how she could do that, but I didn't give her a chance to try. I saw an ad in the paper for a maternal-child nurse at Lovelace-Bataan.

Bob was working there at the time, so I asked him if he minded if I were to work in the same place. He said it was up to me. So, I interviewed and landed the job, choosing to work on the postpartum unit rather than pediatrics. So, I gave my two-week notice and, even on my last day while I was giving the night nurse report, I still did not have the courage to express my anger. I had reported that one of our C-sections had a Foley catheter in. A couple of minutes later, she flipped back the Kardex to that lady's and accused me of not having reported that the lady had a Foley. I felt like saying, "Yes. I did. Weren't you listening, you bitch?" But I didn't have the courage, so I just gritted my teeth and continued with the report. It wouldn't have mattered a hoot since it was my last night, but I just couldn't do it. This, I feel, began a slow fuse burning inside me.

So, in March of 1980, I began working at Lovelace. Things were better, but not perfect. I was doing well in my work and with my peers. However, working with the doctors was a problem for most of the nurses and even the head nurse. As one of the nurses put it, "They are such prima donnas." I was able to defend my position with Dr. Spencer but was not able to express my anger towards Dr. Meinhart. I felt he could have me fired if I opposed his view, and he probably would have. I once told him that the incision of one of his C-section patients was infected and he belittled me by saying that it was a hematoma and asked if I couldn't tell the difference between a hematoma and a wound infection. Of course, I was right but was not about to argue about it. I got around him by reporting it to the resident who took it on his own to lance it and prescribe antibiotics. But with Dr. Spencer, it was somewhat different because if he was wrong, he would come back later and apologize. He once accused me of delaying a lady for surgery in our unit. I yelled right back that we had only had her in our unit for five minutes and that she was pre-opted and was on her way to surgery. So, on January 4th,

1981, all the accumulated and pent-up frustrations exploded in the form of a seizure resulting from the brain tumor.

Another contributing factor, I felt, was that I had been on and off birth control pills in an effort to control the excessive bleeding I had during my menstrual periods, during this time.[25] The reason I felt that the additional hormones contributed to the cause was that I did not feel terribly depressed. I felt more frustrated than depressed or despaired, and I had hope that, once Dr. Spencer arrived, the situation with the doctors would improve. I reasoned that, if certain hormonal changes were responsible for suppressing the immune system, the addition of more hormones could only further upset the hormonal balance in my body, thereby increasing the immunosuppressant effect. [26]

So, the first three weeks of February I spent packing, reading, and I had started learning to meditate although the book advised against starting before the whole book was read. I felt an immediate urgency to do something to help myself and felt it could do no harm to learn to meditate since many people meditate for many reasons whether ill or not.

On February 11th, Tami from the Cancer Center called me to tell me they had scheduled me for a CAT scan in Los Alamos, for Saturday, February 21st at 9 and I was to be at the airport at 7 am. They said they had to have a CAT scan done there so they could compare successive pictures.

By the fourteenth, all the linens except what we had to use, all the books, pictures, collectibles, knick-knacks, toys, and most of the dishes were packed. Bob had made arrangements with his dad and sister to come down and help him drive. I had made arrangements to stay with Katie for two weeks while I awaited the trip to Los Alamos.

I decided I had to say goodbye to the girls at Lovelace. So, Friday, I left the kids with Bob and went to Lovelace. I went up to the

---

[25] Birth control pills can have an impact on cardiovascular disease; however, they have no link to brain tumors. In fact, birth control pills can be protective against ovarian cancer.

[26] There is no clinical evidence to support a role for birth control in promoting tumors or creating a change in immune surveillance of the brain.

fourth floor. I told them that we were moving to Wisconsin, but I had to stay in New Mexico to take the treatments in Los Alamos. I relayed to them that I was a bit hesitant about doing this as it would be pretty lonely not to be able to see Bob for seven weeks. The consolation would be, I informed them, that I was keeping Karen with me. They said it would be like having your man out to sea when in the service. The girls wished me luck and said to drop in when I was in Albuquerque for the weekends. I told them that I would, depending on whether or not I would have to stay in Los Alamos for the weekend. I was told they would run the treatments from Monday through Friday, but if the machine should break down, it would be necessary to do them on the weekend. As I left, they hugged me. I left feeling that I might be missed after all.

I went out to the floor to say bye to the rest of the staff. Elaine, a nursing assistant, who liked me very much, insisted that I write to her once I got to Wisconsin. I was not as fond of her as she was of me, but I told her I would write, probably not to each of them personally, but to the whole staff. Once I got to La Crosse, however, my problems became so consuming that I didn't even think of writing and when I did, I was too tired to do it.

I was so grateful to the people that had helped me during my illness, that I felt indebted to them in some small way. In my heart, I felt that I should return their love and concern in some small way. I especially wanted to do something nice for Sally since she had taken on a great burden. The least was expected of her since, in this day and age [and] in most communities, good neighbors are hard to find.

I knew I wasn't going to be around to return a favor for these people but did not find it difficult to know what I was going to get them. I'd spend hours, (though not at one time) watching Ann paint crystal balls for Christmas ornaments while I was helping out in the nursery, and the babies were sleeping or out to their mothers. Admiringly, I'd sit in the nurses' station which divided the two nurseries, watching her paint while I wished I only had a fraction of her talent. So, after I gave the rest of the staff my farewell, I went down the hall to see Ann. I asked her how much she charged for the balls and whether she had any left after Christmas. She said she charged $11 for the big ones and $9 for the little ones, justifying the high price by saying that she charged that much because she had put so much time into them. I told her I understood and did not think the price was unreasonably high as stores charged that and more for ordinary ones and hers were beautiful. She said she had four left and that I could drop by after work to see them. She gave me directions to her house.

So Friday at three, I set out to Ann's house, taking the kids with me as Bob had already gone to work. When I got there, she showed me what she had and what she could sell me. I chose one with a lantern by a window and holly scene, another large one with a hearth scene, and a small one with an angel scene. I wanted to give one to Mom and one to Sally since they had helped me so much. They were so beautiful that I wanted one for myself also. They were very delicate frosted glass crystal balls, which she painted. The painting required a definite finesse since the many lines were so fine. I paid her for the three balls. As I was leaving, she said something about having to go to her jazzercise class. Offhand, I said, "I ought to join too. Would you believe that I gained weight in the hospital? I would like to just get down to where my clothes aren't tight." She said, "That's the nice thing about exercise. You can weigh a little more and your clothes still fit." I never forgot what she said.

Actually, that's when I began thinking that I would like to join a jazzercise class. I was never very athletic but always liked dancing. So, it would be [the] perfect exercise for me. What got me thinking about exercise was *Getting Well Again*. It advocated exercise as part of the program to recovery. They had noticed a positive correlation between vigorous physical exercise and patients who were most successfully treated. The theory behind exercise being beneficial is that exercise causes lymphocytosis, stimulating the immune system to fight the cancer cells.

Another person I wanted to give special thanks to was Katie. She hadn't babysat or fixed meals, but she was always there when I needed her. Next to Bob, she gave me the greatest emotional support. I didn't get her a ball because I thought she would really like a cowboy hat since she had admired mine so when she saw it. So, I called Katie on Saturday and asked her if she would like to go shopping with me. We always had fun when we were shopping since our tastes were so similar. So, she agreed, and I told her I'd pick her up in an hour.

When I arrived at her house, she was still getting ready but that didn't matter; it gave us more time to chat. While she was occupied in the other room, I would read *Rocky Mountain Magazine* or some of the other professional journals that she had laying on the handsome pine coffee table they had recently bought. She usually offered me a coke and I usually accepted.

When we left, the dogs beat us to the door, especially Rastus, he loved to get away and run. But we managed to keep him in and get out of the house and into my car. When in the car, I told Katie that I wanted to buy her something in appreciation for what she had done for me. She said, "Oh you don't have to." I said, "No, but I want to." I asked her where she wanted to go. She said that she didn't care, and I didn't either, so we ended up at Coronado Center. We were in no hurry, so we browsed. When we got to Goldwater's, we went to the hat section. Katie tried on a number of different hats, most of them being too big. She commented about having a small head. But she finally found one that she really liked. It was a really nice straw cowboy hat. I told her I'd buy it for her. She looked at the price tag and asked, "Are you sure?"

"Sure, after all you've done for me, I want you to have something nice." After some coaxing, she accepted. It was still a little big, but the sales lady referred us to a place where we could get a spongy filler that you place between the trim on the inside of the hat. She also gave us two hat boxes, although I had bought mine several weeks before. We went to the leather shop to which she had referred us, and we both got our hats adjusted. I was surprised that he didn't charge us anything. We had lunch at Vip's Big Boy and then left for home.

As our move was fairly unexpected, it turned out to be a big free-for-all. I had already given most of my baby equipment and accessories to Katie, but there were odd pieces of furniture that weren't really worth taking along, so Bob decided to get rid of them. Karen had been sleeping on a small, low vinyl studio couch-type bed with a mattress on top. It was placed in a corner at a right angle next to the other identical bed. It had a four-legged white square table that stood over the end of the other bed. We had covered the table with contact paper with forest scenery with rabbits and squirrels and bear cubs, typical nursery style. We gave that to Katie and Dave. Karen also gave her two dolls, "so she could have a baby while she waited for hers." She also gave Katie her own little yellow and white crocheted infant dress.

There were a couple of end tables with unstable legs and marred surfaces that were not worth anything, and Bob thought that no one would want them, so he put them out on the driveway so that the garbage men could pick them up. But Jim, our neighbor, came over and asked Bob if he could have them. Bob told him that he could, offered him a beer, and gave him other miscellaneous things that we were not going to take to Wisconsin. His son, Jack, inherited the Legos as Bob did not intend to take toys that would get lost anyway, and Ken just did not have the interest in them that Jack did.

Bob's dad and sister, Lisa, arrived on the eighteenth (Jan. 18th). They had flown in on a one-way ticket as they were going to help Bob drive back. Bob went to pick them up at the airport. When they came through the front door, the kids went wild with joy, jumping up and down in their excitement and yelling, "Grandpa, Grandpa, Lisa, Lisa." They loved [both] their grandfather and their aunt. Hugs and kisses were exchanged, but we soon had to resume packing as there was still much work to be done. The original moving plan was that Bob and his Dad would pack everything, including the beds, and that they would sleep in sleeping bags in the house. Lisa and Karen would spend the night at Katie's and set out the next day.

Bob and Dad packed all the tools in the garage, which was a big job, and took the rest of the day as Bob had accumulated a lot in the first 10 years of our marriage. He also had made a corner desk that we had used in the apartment when we were going to school, and he had used it for a workshop table in the garage while we lived in the house on Wellesley.

The next day, Bob made arrangements to put up the house for sale. He contacted a friend's mother, a realtor, whom he felt had our best interests in mind when selling the house. She came to the house, measured it inside and out, listed its assets and we settled on an asking price of $60,000. Bob had also asked me whether or not we should take Wilbur, our St. Bernard. "Of course, we'll have to take him," I pleaded. I couldn't believe he could have thought of leaving him behind. "We can't just get rid of him after six years. We're the only owners he's had."

"That's what I thought," he said, "I just had to be sure." I had started packing my personal things from the bathroom when Bob and Dad went to buy paint and other materials they needed to put the house up for sale. I put most everything into my train case and the bigger things into a box. My jewelry went into a plastic bag, in my train case, as Katie had advised that I keep that with me.

I had seen most of my friends and bid them goodbye, but I had not seen Jennifer. She and I had shared some of the frustrations of working for male-chauvinistic doctors. I had to see her one last time before I left. So, I gave her a call. She said I could drop by about one. So, I made a quick lunch for Bob and Dad. Lisa was having lunch and reminiscing with some of her old Albuquerque friends. Ken felt big and important helping Grandpa and Dad, and Lisa had taken Karen with her. So, I told the guys that I wanted to visit a special friend and I'd be back later to continue working.

So, I went to Jennifer's house by myself. She had just had a baby, a boy this time, whom she was nursing. We talked about babies of course, usually the subject to talk about when there's a baby around. She said she'd had a terrible labor this time as compared to the last time when she had a premature baby girl. A seven-pound boy made quite a difference, but she was consoled by the fact that her nurse-midwife stayed with her throughout the labor. She also said that this baby was very fussy as compared to her little girl and that she was going to give [him] a pacifier any time he wanted to keep him quiet. I asked her if she had tried a baby swing, because Karen had been fussy as an infant and the swing is where she spent most of the day. She said she had but the baby did not even like that.

Then, we talked about how our lives would be in the next few years. She thought I was lucky to be going to Wisconsin, she'd heard it was beautiful. I had my reservations about it, but that maybe it would be a new start. She said that her husband was thinking of doing a residency in one of the Northwestern states.

When I got home, I resumed the work cleaning the sinks, toilets, bathtub, and shower stall. The shower stall took the longest, but I also took a shower while I was in there. The grooves between the tiles were small and tended to mildew easily. I had to take an old toothbrush and scrub away. I also vacuumed the bathroom floor to get it ready to be scrubbed.

Bob and I had taken the plants down. I had them hanging on cute macramé hangers that I had made by the west window. Actually, I took the plants down and put some of the healthier ones in open boxes to take to Wisconsin, and he took down the platform "grow lights" above them, as Bob called them. He had bought them as our plants did not get much sunlight on the west window.

Dad packed everything, even a few useless things such as old grocery bags. He did not want to be accused of not packing something we wanted.

"You'd even pack the trash," I teased.

"You bet," he laughed. Then, he went on to explain that professional packers did pack the trash if it was around, lest they be accused of stealing.

On the morning of the nineteenth, Bob ordered a U-Haul truck, and he and his Dad went to pick it up. As soon as they arrived, they began loading it, beginning with the big pieces of furniture and large appliances.

Lisa and I cleaned and scrubbed the bathrooms getting on our hands and knees to scrub the dirt and wax build-up off the floors. Lisa kept repeating, "I never thought I'd be on my hands and knees scrubbing floors."

It was drawing close to lunchtime, and I was rummaging through the refrigerator and shelves to see what I might put together for lunch to use up what we had before we actually moved, when the phone rang. It was Tami, from the Cancer Center. She called to remind me to be at the airport at seven and then she said, "Oh, be prepared to have your head shaved." I was shocked and in desperation, I asked, "All of it?"

"Yes," she replied.

"Well, you can take your program and stuff it," I retorted, angrily.

"Well, if it's not for you, it's not for you," she answered in a stunned voice.

My father-in-law had been putting canned goods in a box when he heard me tell her off. His eyes widened and his jaw dropped, in amazement as he had never heard me talk to anyone like that. His look of surprise turned into a grin. Lisa had been cleaning the shelves above the laundry area and she smiled and said, "Right on! You told them."

I hung up the phone and remarked, "Well I guess I'm going with you." Bob came in from the garage a few seconds later. I told him what had happened. "Bet you're glad," I said. He was overjoyed. He hugged me. He didn't think he could survive seven weeks without some nookie. He was also worried that I'd get interested in some doctor or psychologist while he was gone.

While we had a smorgasbord of leftovers, I made arrangements for a change of itinerary. I was sitting on the blue swivel chair amidst a clutter of boxes in which kitchen utensils, food, and other paraphernalia lay. I looked out the kitchen window with a sigh. I gazed out of the window and for a few moments just stared. It was [a] cool, breezy overcast day, but last spring I'd finally had some success in landscaping. I had three-square surfaces on which I had planted flowers. I had also planted vines and rose bushes along the trellises. Bob had put up the trellis at right angles to each other and left about a foot around them for flowers. I wasn't aware of what I was staring at, but at an unconscious level, I knew I'd miss this house.

Bob snapped me out of my daydream by mentioning, "Guess you'll have to notify a lot of people of your change in plans."

"Huh- oh- yeah. Mom already took the time off to be with me, I had the hospital send the disability payments to Katie's house and gave them her number at the cancer center. I'll have to tell Katie I won't be spending two weeks with her and of course Dr. Golden."

"You'll have to have the hospital send your records to La Crosse."

So, I spent the next half hour on the phone. I called Dr. Golden, saying, "I'm sorry that I put you through all that trouble, but I've decided to go to La Crosse with Bob after all. He asked me what made me change my mind. Being truthful, I explained that I could not bear the thought of them shaving all of my hair off. He referred me to Dr. Anderson at the Gundersen Clinic, instructing me to send my records to the clinic but to go down to the record room myself because if I phoned in, it would probably not get done.

I called Mom who was more understanding when I told her that I would be going with Bob and the kids, but I noticed a sadness in her voice as she reminded me that she had already taken the time off. Perhaps I heard a note of regret that she could not do one more thing for me. I persisted in saying, "But you can go back if you want to; can't you?" She said that she could. I sensed an air of concern and solemnity being transmitted through the phone, as I said "I'll be okay, Mom. I'll call when we get there."

I went to the hospital in order to release my records. I was directed to the basement of the hospital where medical records are kept. I wandered around the basement until I found the Medical Record Department. There was a small woman in a red dress sitting behind a small desk with spectacles on. She stood up as I approached the desk and asked what she could do for me. I gave the woman my name and told her that I wanted my records released to the Gundersen Clinic in La Crosse. She asked me which doctor they were to be released to. I told her that I didn't remember but it started with an A. Then she asked me who my doctor was, and I told her Dr. Golden. She told me she would contact his office and find out, meanwhile, to have a seat while she looked for my chart. After waiting at the chair beside her desk, I was beginning to get bored and wondering why it should take so long to find a chart. Finally, she came back to her desk, saying she couldn't find it. So, she made several phone calls and finally discovered that my chart was at the Cancer Center. She told me that if I signed the two release forms, she'd make sure they got to La Crosse. I had no reason to doubt her, so I signed them and went on my way.

Bob, Dad, and Ken were going to leave on the twentieth. Lisa volunteered to stay an extra day to help me drive and also to have one last fling with her friends from Lovelace. Lisa had already packed a separate grocery box for me to take to Los Alamos. She had packed canned and dried goods, things that wouldn't spoil while I bid my time at Katie's. I was actually looking forward to spending a little time with Katie. But the food became unnecessary when I changed my plans, so she began to unpack one box and repack them with the other foods. We did have some items that would spoil, like milk that I put in that box and ran over to Sally's house.

I had packed a suitcase full of sweaters and pants. I had heard that Los Alamos was cold this time of year. I had also packed two small suitcases for Karen. Lisa was a bit miffed at me for wanting to put Karen's and my suitcases in the Pinto, which she would not even try to put hers in. She resentfully threw her suitcase into the truck that Bob and Dad were packing. Little did she know that, if it did not fit, I would be willing to put one of Karen's in the truck.

CHAPTER 7

The morning of the twentieth was a busy one. Bob and his Dad went to pick up a large rental moving truck. Once they got moving, they really got moving. All the big furniture was put in the truck first. The beds were disassembled, and the mattresses were used as padding between furniture to prevent marring. Even Karen's beanbag chair was used for that purpose. Next to be loaded were the many boxes of books, records, knick-knacks, and pictures. After that, more boxes of linens and small kitchen appliances were loaded. Next were the toys. Even though Bob had eliminated what he thought was unnecessary, there were still many toys to load. I had put most of them in Ken's toy chest that his great-uncle had made for him. They were merely boxes made of plywood stacked on top of one another and painted red, yellow, and blue—all colors Ken had chosen. Most of the toys fit in there. But, of course, we couldn't leave behind the boxes Ken and I had made for Karen. They were fiberfill boxes that I picked up at Allwoods. She had picked softer colors for us to paint them, a pastel blue and green. They were small and she used them mostly as bookshelves. But she treasured them as Kenny had made them for her. She also could not leave her little kitchen that she had received for her birthday. It was not so little and did take up some room in the truck, but I had packed it with her storybooks, so it did its job. More boxes of dishes and canned goods came next. The last thing to be put in the truck was the refrigerator and freezer. We kept the freezer full. It was felt that if they traveled straight through for twenty-eight hours, that there was sufficient coldness to keep the food frozen. The house was completely empty by 2 p.m., and rather than stay the night in the sleeping bags as they had planned, they decided to take off right then. Lisa had taken Karen with her to see some of her friends, so she had my car, and I was stuck in the empty house to wait for the carpet cleaners to come.

I was a little miffed over this, and I said, "Thanks a lot guys. Just leave me alone with no car, nothing to sit on, and no music or television to watch."

Bob replied, "Well, someone has to let the carpet cleaners in." I probably would have volunteered anyway but I was a little teed off at being taken for granted.

But it was a good time to get some reading done on my book. Still, I felt resentful over being left alone in an empty [and] uncomfortable house. The steam cleaners for the rug came and cleaned the rug while I went out to the yard to read. When they left, the rug was still wet so I couldn't even stretch out on my belly and read in a more comfortable position, so I picked the driest spot I could find, sat down, and leaned against the wall. I was still worried about just how much of my tumor remained and just how much was Grade 3, and how that would affect my life. Being alone in an empty house only increased my anxiety and frustration. Being alone with my thoughts at this time was not very productive, yet I knew I had to quit feeling sorry for myself because, as the book says, those kinds of feelings contribute to the suppression of the immune system, which in turn allows abnormal cells to survive.[27]

Finally, about four o'clock, Lisa came back with my car, and we set out to Katie's house. Katie, Dave, Karen, and I had supper at their house. Katie had invited Lisa too, but she refused, saying that she and her friends had plans for an evening at one of their favorite restaurants.

Karen was cooperative but worried that she and I were going to Los Alamos instead of Wisconsin even though we had reassured her that I had changed my plans and we were following Dad and

---

27 There is no evidence that "feelings" contribute to immune suppression or survival of abnormal cells.

Ken to Wisconsin. The fact that Daddy and Ken left before us proved in her mind that we were not going to Wisconsin. She slept with me that night.

After supper, I helped Katie with the dishes. Then, we watched a little television and talked, mostly reminiscing over past good times and how I wished that I could be there when her baby arrived. I had already informed her of our changed plans, but she said, "I was looking forward to your staying here."

"So was I," I admitted. "We'll be back for summers, though."

"Yeah, and we'd like to see that part of the country. We can't go this year, but we can probably make it in two years."

Dave had gone with Bob, Dad, and Ken to help drive as he was out of work anyway, and they sure could use the help driving since they were taking two vehicles, a rental moving truck, and the van. While the truck held most of our earthly possessions, there was not much in the van other than Wilbur and some of my plants. A two-hundred-pound St. Bernard takes a lot of room even in the back of a van. Their plan was that two could drive while one slept. They knew that no motel would allow a St. Bernard, so they planned to drive straight through. Ken switched back and forth from the truck to the van.

Meanwhile, Katie and I continued to chat, reminisce, and plan for future vacations when we could see one another again. Although nothing was said, we mutually knew we would miss each other. I had put Karen to bed and had left a closet light on as her night light was probably in the truck. Finally, about eleven o'clock, I decided to retire, since we were to start out early the next morning. She understood and said she'd stay up to let Lisa in.

We said goodnight, and I climbed into bed with Karen. She cuddled while sleeping but also kicked during the night, but I didn't mind because my anxiety was still high, and her warm body was a source of comfort for me.

Katie fell asleep on the sofa waiting to let Lisa in. I'm a light sleeper so I heard the knocking on the door. I waited a while since Katie said she'd let her in, and I was still very drowsy. The knocking continued for a while, and just as I was about to get up and open the door, I heard Katie open it and say something to Lisa. I looked up at the lighted alarm clock and saw it was 3 a.m. "Great," I thought, "She'll be in <u>fine</u> shape for driving!"

We got up at 6:30 to be on the road by seven. Katie offered us breakfast, but I refused saying we could stop on the way as I was never hungry that early, anyway. Lisa refused also. Karen was asleep, and we carried her into the car. We put our suitcases in the car and came back in to say goodbye. Katie and I hugged each other.

She said, "I'm going to miss you."

It was hard for me to say goodbye, and all I managed to say was, "Me, too."

I told Lisa that I would drive first so that she could get some sleep. She slept for about an hour, then Karen woke up and when she was fully awake, she was excited to be going and kept trying to get Lisa to play with her as she had done on previous trips. Only, Karen didn't find Lisa so delightful this time. Lisa kept saying, "Stop that, Karen. I'm trying to get some sleep." They finally both went to sleep about ten o'clock so I drove on without stopping for a break. We had packed some snacks, which I munched on.

I drove until it was getting close to lunchtime. By this time, I was feeling really sick. We stopped by a gas station bathroom, but since we didn't need gas, we stopped in a parking lot next to the gas station. I didn't make it to the bathroom and vomited in the parking lot. I went into the bathroom, which happened to be open, but I only retched and retched. My stomach was empty, but my brain wouldn't believe it. It was also that time of the month, and I had cramps, which probably explained why I was feeling so ill. But here we were, out in the middle of nowhere, close to Tucumcari, NM but I knew no one there, and I was only six weeks post-op, so I panicked. The Tegretol overdose was still very much on my mind, and I didn't know whether I should call my doctor or what. I asked Lisa what I should do, try to call my doctor, or just wait and see. It was foolish to ask her as she was still young and inexperienced, so naturally, she said, "I don't know; whatever you think." There was a phone booth in the parking lot, and I got as far as picking up the receiver, but my nausea was starting to subside, and I noticed the park across the street, so I put the receiver back, came out of the booth, and told Lisa, "Why don't we go rest in that park?" I must have looked pretty green, as she seemed to be a bit frightened, so I said (mostly to reassure her) that we should get some soda and go to the park. I could rest and Karen could swing, and it probably was just due to my period anyway, that I just got frightened, since we were far away from home.

The park across the street from the parking lot had a small playground with swings and brightly painted jump animals, which could entertain Karen while I rested. It was not a very cold February afternoon, the dew had already evaporated, and so I just lay on the grass with my jacket on. My eyes felt heavy, and the fresh air smelled sweet in this small-unpolluted town. I dozed, or nearly dozed, but I did not let myself go completely asleep, as I knew Lisa wanted to get back quickly because she had to go to work Monday morning. I got up in about an hour, telling Lisa that I felt better but still not well enough to eat, but if she and Karen wanted to stop somewhere to eat, that was fine with me. Lisa said that she was on a diet anyway and Karen was still anxious to catch up with Daddy and Ken. So, we drove on with Karen snacking on the things we had brought.

Naturally, Lisa drove the rest of the day since I'd been feeling ill. She drove well into the evening. I suggested stopping for something to eat as none of us had really eaten that day. We stopped at a small café, the kind with the turnstile jukebox speaker at your booth to which you insert a quarter for three songs. We didn't play it, but Karen flipped the keys. We were seated in the first booth near the door. I ordered a grilled cheese sandwich for Karen and a bowl of homemade vegetable soup for myself, as I didn't want to put anything heavy in my stomach yet. Lisa ordered a cheeseburger.

After we ate, Lisa continued to drive. She kept on driving until about ten, and I think she intended to drive straight through. But I knew she had not had much sleep the previous night. She might have done all right by herself, but I had the responsibility of thinking of Karen and myself. So, I tried to tactfully suggest that we find a place for the night. She was a little peeved with my suggestion and suddenly stopped at the first motel she saw.

The motel she stopped at was a really dumpy one at the edge of a small village. She pulled up to the drive-up port and I went into the office. I had never registered at a motel before and was surprised at the amount of information required of you to only spend the night. I didn't know the car's license plate number, so I had to go out and look. The office was a small office, dimly lit, with an older woman sitting behind the counter. I was a little leery about this place but didn't want to argue with Lisa, so I wrote the woman a check for $14 and determined that I would be sure to lock the door. The elderly woman gave me the key and we drove up to the door. Lisa opened the trunk and asked me if we were going to take anything in. I told her I'd need my nightgown and took my suitcase in. The room was a small one with two double beds. There were old dark green and grey floral curtains, the kind you might expect an elderly lady to decorate with. Upon entering the room, I noticed that there wasn't a phone or a television; not that we needed them, nor did I expect any for $14, but it just convinced me that this was a cheap hotel. It reminded me of the kind of motel room on television shows where the murder takes place. So as soon as everyone was in, I locked both the door and the bolt lock.

I commented, "This sure is a creepy place; it gives me that eerie feeling."

Lisa added, "Well you said to stop." I said nothing more, and Lisa went into the bathroom.

I asked Karen who she wanted to sleep with and she said Lisa. I was a bit disappointed and tried not to show it. It was still a fearful time for me, and if I could not have Bob next to my side, I'd settle for her. But I didn't argue.

While Lisa was in the bathroom and Karen was on her bed falling asleep, I decided to meditate. I fluffed up the pillow and put it lengthwise against the headboard to lean back on, then began to relax. I began to relax by starting with my facial muscles, continuing on downwards until I reached the tips of my toes. When I was completely relaxed, I began to imagine what I wanted: the rest of my tumor to be gone. To do that I needed a symbol (as the book suggested). I chose sharks because the book said that they were the most successful. So, I imagined the sharks coming from every part of my body, working their way up to my brain and eating up that tumor.

When Lisa returned from the bathroom, I quickly washed up and brushed my teeth, then went to bed but did not immediately go to sleep. The sharks were still swimming around in my mind.

As there was no phone service, Lisa was glad she had brought a little wind-up alarm clock, so we could get an early start the next day. She set the alarm for five, and we were on the road by six. It was still dark when we left and, fortunately, Karen was still sleeping. I carried her to the car, letting her sleep on my lap. The Pinto did not have enough space, even to let a child sleep comfortably, and we wanted her to sleep as long as possible. So, Lisa drove first. Lisa put the suitcase and train case in the car, which I thanked her for.

Lisa continued to drive until lunchtime when Karen began to get hungry. We stopped at a restaurant right off the highway, so we could get on the road again. It was a family-type restaurant, and we ordered nothing fancy, just hamburgers and a strawberry shake for Karen.

We made it to Kansas City about 3 p.m. that afternoon. I wanted to see my sister Carol. And before I left, she had insisted that I stop at her place, I presume to see for herself that I was all right. Since Lisa had been driving, I tried to give her directions from my half-forgotten memory of where she lived. I knew we were supposed to get on Interstate 475, but we just passed it as I saw it, and had no time to tell Lisa to stop and get off. So, we got off at the next exit, reversed directions, and tried to locate the entry ramp to I475. But it turned out to be useless. Wherever this exit had led us, it was nowhere near the last exit. After driving around for about an hour with our nerves getting on edge, I suggested we stop at a little grocery store near where we were and ask for directions to the freeway.

Lisa was disgruntled and said, "I'm not going to ask!"

I've never been embarrassed about asking for directions, so I said, "I will." (My sense of direction was never good, and I often got lost.) The directions were not the clearest, and neither of us knew the city or the landmarks, so the first time we tried to follow them we drove around the block. In frustration, Lisa said, "I can't follow directions that someone else took." I said, "Okay, I'll drive, you read them to me." As following the first directions only took us around the block, I decided that one of the landmarks was either wrong or that there had to be another one similar to it. So instead [of turning at [the] designated spot that took us around the block, I went all the way down the street and then followed the directions. That got us close enough to find the interstate again. A little more driving got us to the interstate. Lisa was on the lookout for the right exit and, this time, we got off at the right one. The exit led us all the way across Kansas City to the Missouri side, where Carol and Ben lived. This time, my memory was clearer, and I got off on the right exit. I recognized the shopping center near the turnoff that was one landmark to her house, but I couldn't remember where to go from there. There was also now a new major department store in addition to the shopping center on the other side of the street, which only served to confuse me more. I decided to pull into the parking lot of the shopping center, which had a phone booth. I went to the phone booth, looked up Carol's phone number, and called her. She said we were close and gave me further directions to the street she lived on and said that I'd be able to find it from there. What she didn't realize was that brain surgery could affect your memory and that it had been over a year since I'd been there. So, we found the street with no problem, but I didn't remember which house it was and had forgotten to write the address down from the phone book. So, in my dimmed memory, I thought it was the second or third house on the street. What I didn't remember was that the street turned into a cul-de-sac at the end of the street and that it was the second house on the cul-de-sac. I stopped at the second house on the street and told Lisa to wait in the car as I wasn't sure it was the right house. I rang the bell, and a young woman of medium stature and light brown hair answered. I asked if she knew where the Jakes lived. She had no idea, so she asked her husband who also had no idea. So, I went back to the car and tried to rack my brain to remember what her house looked like and where on the street it was, but it was hopeless. Meanwhile, Ben, her husband, showed up, recognized us, and escorted us to his house.

We greeted each other, and when Ben told her where he had found us, she said, "I was sure you'd remember where our house was."

I just smiled and said, "It's been a long time." I was embarrassed to admit that the brain surgery might have affected my memory.

Ben then excused himself saying he had to go buy some materials for his dental school project. After he left, we sat around and talked for an hour, mostly about my surgery and some about our trip. I suggested that we leave, as I knew Lisa was upset about the delay I had caused by wanting to see Carol and not knowing exactly where she lived. Carol invited us for supper, insisting that we stay at least until Ben came back since he hardly had a chance to see us. She really wanted us to stay, but she was wondering when Ben would be home as he said he'd only be a few minutes.

I was doubtful as to whether Lisa wanted to stay or not, so I turned to her and said, "Well what do you think?"

"We're already here," she acquiesced.

Ben returned about six o'clock. Carol was just putting the finishing touches on her dinner. She put plates out for Lisa and me to set out. Ben grabbed a handful of mismatching silverware, whereupon Carol reproached him. Lisa and I said it didn't matter. We weren't company, only family. She responded by saying, "Well, Ben knows how his family appreciates fine silverware." Ben couldn't have cared less about whether the silverware matched as his smirked grin let us know. But he said not a word to her.

After dinner, Lisa and I helped clear the table, but she would not let us help with the dishes, as she preferred to rinse the dishes in the sink before putting them in the dishwasher. As it was after seven when dishes were done, and there would be only a few hours left of driving, we decided to spend the night there. Karen and I used the guest bedroom, and Lisa slept on the couch.

Again, we got up early to get an early start. Carol would have preferred that we stayed since it was Sunday and she could have taken us to some interesting places in Kansas City, but Lisa had to go to work the next day, so it was imperative to leave now.

Lisa drove until early afternoon when we reached Iowa. It was a cold cloudy day with the sky getting darker as we drove on. As we reached Iowa, little white crystals began to decorate our windshield. As she drove further, the snow began to get thicker.

My concern was that the roads would get slicker if this persisted or got worse, so I asked Lisa to let me drive. So, she stopped the car, and we switched places. It continued to lightly snow until we were almost out of Iowa and then it stopped. Lisa let me drive until we got to Cedar Rapids, where she wanted to drive because from there she said she knew a shortcut. I didn't object as I was getting tired.

Karen had been pretty good throughout the long trip since we hadn't made many stops, but as toys and car games became boring, she decided to talk on the CB. Lisa and I didn't object, as long as it kept her happy. She was just happily chatting, pretending to talk to Bo and Luke Duke, when an irritated trucker came over the CB and cursed her telling her to get off the air in no uncertain terms. I was irritated but it made Lisa mad. She told them, "Hey, I've heard you guys pick up girls over this thing." We left the CB on and didn't hear another word from them.

I wasn't very hungry, but it had been a long drive, and I thought Karen might be hungry or need a pit stop, so around six o'clock, I asked whether anybody wanted to stop and eat. As I thought Karen might be hungry, I asked her, "Do you want to stop at a restaurant and eat or drive all the way to Wisconsin." She kept her persistent attitude and to my surprise, she said that she wanted to go straight to Wisconsin. This put me in a rough stop as I wanted to make a pit stop. But that was the answer that Lisa wanted, and we made no stops. So, we drove for two more hours, and I thought my bladder was going to burst.

We arrived at Grandma and Grandpa's house at about eight that evening. By the time we got there, Lisa had the same problem. We both made a mad dash to the bathroom, but she beat me. Was I ever mad! She had known I had to go for two hours, yet she purposely usurped the bathroom.

"You did that on purpose," I snapped.

She just grinned, "First come, first served."

After the necessities were taken care of, we greeted everyone. I was glad to see Bob. We hugged and kissed, and Karen cut in on the action as she had missed her dad too. Ken greeted me by saying, "Mommy, Mommy," and throwing his arms around me. Karen was overjoyed to see both of them. At last, her family was together.

Mom and Dad were of course glad to see us and were also concerned as to how I felt. I'm sure my surgery was still very much on their minds. But I was not concerned for the moment and just said, "Much better."

Grandma reheated the leftovers and, by that time, all of us were famished. It had been a long day so I wanted to retire as soon as I could get the kids to bed. I had been told by Dad, Bob, and Dave that Ken had behaved great on the trip and even that day before I arrived. Grandpa did tell me that the only naughty thing he had done on the trip was throwing baby powder all over the cab of the truck while [Grandpa] was gassing up. But when I told him to go to bed that night, he resisted, yelling at me that he didn't have to.

I was hurt and responded, "Real nice, you're real good when I'm gone but you start acting up the minute I return! Do you know how that makes me feel?" I asked angrily. There seemed to be some kind of chemistry between us that didn't jive, or maybe he was reacting as younger children do when their mothers leave them for the day. But I hadn't left him. They had left ahead of us. I just didn't understand and was perhaps a little jealous that he behaved better for others than he did for me. "Why did he have to treat me like that?" I thought.

In the meantime, I heard Bob say, "Is that any way to treat your mother? Mind your mother, and get your pajamas on!"

Karen played with Ken a little that evening and sat on Daddy's lap playing with and teasing him. Lisa had left hurriedly, after grabbing a bite to eat, as she had to do laundry before going to work in the morning. However, it was not hard to put Karen to bed that night as she was tired. She fell asleep on the sofa and Bob carried her up to the bedroom.

We talked a bit after that. They mentioned the events of their trip, including the one where Grandpa, Bob, and Dave ordered hamburgers and Ken ordered shrimp. My in-laws were also concerned about how I felt. There was not much to tell about our trip, although I did mention the motel. Bob asked me how much we paid to stay there. When I answered $14, he said, "That <u>was</u> a cheap motel." I was tired and retired shortly after that.

CHAPTER 8

The next three days were busy ones. We had to find a place to live either big enough to store our belongings or an apartment and a storage locker for our things. The truck had to be returned on the 25th of February.

We spent the 23rd and 24th looking for an apartment. Bob, Dave, and I started out early Monday morning and headed for La Crosse. My first introduction to Wisconsin weather was a sharp, knife-like cutting wind that went right through my heavy leather coat to my bones. Bob parked the van in front of a listing bureau-an agency that lists house[s] and apartments for rent or sale, price, and description of the premises.

The listing bureau was on a corner lot. When we got out of the car, we saw a desk with a woman behind it and a door behind the desk that led to another room. Directly behind the desk were grey metal cabinets with many folders of housing available in La Crosse, I presume. Bob told her what we were looking for, and she handed him three books. We looked through the books trying to find a three-bedroom house or apartment that would allow children. Wilbur would stay on the farm until we could buy a house of our own. There was a counter all around the wall in that room with telephones so that we could call the places we wanted to visit. I thought it was pretty cold in the building and kept my coat on until I warmed up. The counter was along a large glass window panel, which I'm sure contributed to the heat loss in the building.

Bob was looking for a house or apartment with reasonable rates since we would be paying rent in La Crosse and a house payment in Albuquerque. Bob wrote some addresses down, and we went to see them. Most of them had something wrong with them. Unfortunately, most of the listings that sounded ideal were in French Island, a section of town that Bob refused to rent in because he said we'd probably be flooded out. The morning was spent looking at about three houses. The one Bob and Dave decided was the best house for the money was a small, economical three-bedroom house with one bath and a medium-sized kitchen.

Dave said, "For the money, this one's your best bet." Bob agreed with him.

"And how are we going to get our bed in here, much less the rest of our bedroom furniture," I asked sarcastically. I was not trying to be extravagant as they may have thought, but I was trying to be practical. Bob took a second look at the bedroom and realized that I was right. So that house was decided against. That took up most of the morning, and we were hungry.

So, we went downtown, and Bob parked in the parking garage, which meant we had to walk a little way to a restaurant. We were headed for a chic little place called Big Al's. While we were walking to the place, I clung to Bob as the icy wind again pierced through to my bones. Even with gloves, my hands were cold, and I'd take them off to blow my warm breath on them. When we entered Big Al's I was relieved. I was still cold, so I kept my coat on until I warmed up a bit. A waitress in a short skirt came up to give us our menus. Bob ordered a beer, and Dave ordered a Stroh's beer, his favorite beer. He wanted to savor his last Stroh's in Wisconsin since it is not sold in New Mexico. While they were drinking their beers and we were scanning the menu, they teased me about being so cold. They said that I'd never make it in Wisconsin if I thought this was cold. I told Bob that the first thing I was buying of the things he promised me was a down snowsuit.

The waitress came back to take our order, and since she had given us plenty of time to decide, the boys ordered another beer. I just ordered a Coke. Bob and I ordered a hero-type sandwich and Dave ordered a pizza sandwich, which turned out to be larger than he expected, but he ate it anyway. The food was good and generous, and we also got potato chips and kosher pickles with the food. Bob gave me his pickle since he doesn't care for them.

Big Al's was an intriguing place. Hanging from the center of the ceiling is a golden-brass colored small airplane. It is an early 1900s American airplane, open in the pit with crossbars on the wings. There were other antiques and pictures of that era along the walls of the room. The charming cozy room was built like a small auditorium with a ground level and two small upper levels. We entered on the ground level, which was surrounded by a small wooden carved railing that looked much like a small fence. There were gateways at each corner of the room for the waitresses to go through when taking orders and delivering food. The tables were small pine tables for two to four people covered with red gingham tablecloths. The kitchen must have been on the upper level which was where the waitresses brought the food.[28]

Other brass items such as old horns, spoons, and other kitchen accessories complemented the airplane. The wallpaper was a black and white old newspaper print. The whole place gave the atmosphere of a romantic yesteryear. We were seated in the middle of the lower floor under the airplane but slightly to the back and to the right, so we had a good view of the airplane. Bob and Dave did most of the talking while we ate as I was enchanted by the place and was looking around at the various antiques and oddities. We finished our lunch, and Dave said we had to find the train station as he was planning to leave as soon as possible. He was running short on money.

Bob offered to pay for lunch as usual, but Dave objected, not wanting to be a freeloader. Bob insisted, saying he would never be able to pay him for what his services were worth in driving and helping. As it was put that way, Dave accepted.

The first day proved to be fruitless. In the afternoon, we went to the train station, which was on the north side of town. It seemed

---

[28] As of 2023, Big Al's in La Crosse is still in operation as a pizza restaurant. It still has a large model airplane in the original store.

to be the poorer side of town with smaller houses and lots needing more repairs than some of those I had seen driving through the Southside and through downtown.

The train station itself was in good condition, though still old-fashioned in mode. The building was long and narrow with a ticket office inside the building on the side of the building where the tracks were located. The benches where people were to wait were of the past generation, consisting of metal frames and wooden slats. The bulletin boards for posting schedules and announcements were encased in wooden boxes with glass windows. These were placed [in] various places around the room along with some material about the history of trains. There were also pictures of old trains and a model of one in the center of the room. While Dave was at the ticket office discussing when the next departure for Chicago was, Bob and I wandered around the room reading the signs and looking at the pictures. It seemed to take a long time to figure [out] a route that would get him to Albuquerque. It turned out the next departure from La Crosse to Chicago was at 3:30 in the morning. As he was short on money and anxious to get back, he bought a ticket. He and Bob joked about how long it would take him to get to Albuquerque with all the stops and delays that were necessary along the way.

Bob said, "Think you'll be there in two weeks?" This was during the period that the federal government was cutting federal spending on rail travel and closing some of the railroad stations.

When Dave came back from the ticket office, he asked us whether we had ever traveled by train. Bob said he had as a kid. And I said I never had except the short ride in Wisconsin on an old train that was really disappointing. He said that it was very enjoyable and "with it", and if we ever had the time and money, we should take a short trip to Chicago.

We visited two more houses that afternoon which were smaller than the others. After that, we decided to quit for the day and went back to my in-law's house for supper. When Bob's mother heard that Dave was leaving that night, she said she was sorry he had to go so soon and tried to persuade him to stay another night. I rescued him by saying that I'd promised Katie to send him back soon.

Before I had left that morning, my mother-in-law had praised Dave saying, "What a nice boy he was." She continued on the next day raving about how nice he was and how she wished he could have stayed longer.

The next day, Bob was anxious to get an early start. He had written down all the addresses of places to check out. I slept as long as I could that morning, not having had much sleep that night. I was still carrying the burden of anxiety that I had developed over my crisis, and it was much worse at night. Also, the Cowdens only had one bathroom, and I wanted to bathe before I went anywhere, so I had to wait my turn. So, I told Bob to leave without me this time. He informed me that we had to get a place to live, or we would have to pay for an extra day for the truck. So, again I told him to go on without me, just to be sure to choose something big enough for our bedroom furniture, especially the bed.

So, I stayed and bathed and did some of our laundry. My mother-in-law decided to come home for lunch. We put together sandwiches and leftovers. I told her that Bob had gone out early so that he could get a head start. She commented again how nice Dave was and how tired Bob must be after taking him to the train station that night. We fed the kids, and she went back to work.

Bob came back shortly after lunch. He said he'd found a place to live on the south side of town. It was located by the Shelby Mall in Sherwood Manor. So, he took me, the kids, and his Dad to go see it. When I saw the building, I assumed it was a one-family house and gasped with astonishment, "That's it!" It looked like a very large modern two-story house with a double garage.

Bob said, "It's a duplex, dear." The man who was to show it to us was already there. We went in to see both apartments. The duplex apartments were basically the same, except the upstairs apartment had an extra bathroom and a sliding glass door near the dining area that opened out onto a deck. They were three-bedroom apartments with bedrooms large for apartment-sized bedrooms. The disadvantage was that the bedrooms were very close together at the end of a small hall. The bathroom was a full bath in front of the master bedroom but did not connect to it. The kitchen was very small but with workable space. It was a U-shaped kitchen with a stove and refrigerator on the east wall, the sink [was] on the north wall, and a breakfast counter peninsula protruded into the room. The breakfast counter could not be used, however, as on the other side of it was just enough space to put our table and four chairs. The living room was large for an apartment being long and narrow and opening into a dining area. The kitchen also had a small pantry on the south wall. Upon entering the apartment was a small coat closet. The only linen closet was a few shelves in the bathroom. We had inspected the upstairs apartment first.

Upon inspecting the downstairs apartment, Bob said, "The only real difference between them is the bathroom. I don't think an extra bathroom is worth an extra $50 a month. Do you?" I nodded in agreement.

While we were walking through the lower apartment, Bob asked, "Well, do you think you could live here for a few months?" I told him that I could and that it was the best we had seen so far. The apartment cost more than we originally intended to pay for rent, but it had the advantage that we could store the furniture and other belongings, which we did not intend to use until we had a more permanent residence. In the double garage, we could store all our belongings and we could use all the space as long as the upstairs apartment remained unrented, and as it turned out it stayed unrented for the time that we were there.

In the garage, there was also a little room with hook-ups for a washer and dryer. So, we hooked up the washer and dryer. There were some shelves along the south wall of the launderette, where some old jars had been left. We also stored my sewing machine there as it was less dirty. There was also an electrical outlet there for the sewing machine, but I only used it once in the time we were there to mend something. The little room was unheated, so I didn't want to spend much time there except to do laundry. Bob paid a $50 deposit and the rent.

The next day was the big moving day. We moved from my in-laws house to the apartment. Most of our possessions were in the truck, so moving from Viroqua to La Crosse was no problem. So, I packed the suitcases in the Pinto and followed them to La Crosse. I was unsure how to get to the apartment since I had not driven there when we inspected it. We did need help in unloading the truck and getting the furniture we were going to use into the apartment. The entryway was an obstacle because when you entered the front door, you had to take a sharp right and immediately descend to the basement to our apartment. The apartment could also be entered from the garage door, which was on the right of the front door as you entered it. Again, Bob's dad was available to help us. The first thing they unloaded was the freezer, but they left that at Bob's folks' house since we had left all the food in there and it needed electricity to keep the food frozen.

Bob and his dad started unloading things into the garage. I took the lighter things that were not packed and the lighter boxes that we were going to use into the apartment. Some of these things consisted of the two stools we had, one that my brother had carved for Bob and one that I had bought at Pier 1 Imports. The lighter boxes included some of the groceries and some of the dishes that I knew would be essential for homemaking. These were wrapped in towels and linens, so I killed two birds with one stone. Our bed was not too much of a problem to take in as it was in pieces, and it was assembled in the apartment. The toughest piece of furniture to get into the apartment was the dresser. It was about six feet wide and three feet high. Bob and Dad decided it would be easier to get it in through the garage door. Inch by inch, they finally got it down the stairs and through the bedroom door. But once that was accomplished, it was downhill from there. Bob thought that the less we brought in the less we would have to move later. So rather than assemble Ken's bed in the apartment he decided that each child could sleep on a mattress on the floor.

This upset Ken greatly and he began to protest loudly. "Why can't we bring in my bed? You're bringing in yours!" He loved the double-decker bed his father had made for him. I tried to console him by telling him he would have his bed back when we sold the house in Albuquerque and bought one in Wisconsin. Bob quickly reproached [Ken's] complaining in a loud, stern manner.

The rest of the furniture that we moved into the apartment was the chest of drawers, the end tables, each of the kid's chest of drawers, our kitchen table and four swivel chairs, the stereo cabinet, the couch, the loveseat, and an easy chair. We also brought in a type of coffee table that could be extended. It was made of interlocking slabs of wood. Everything else, including our large bookshelves, was stored in the garage.

On Friday, February 27th, another cold grey sky morning, Bob and I left the kids with Grandpa and Grandma in order to go to La Crosse to accomplish the necessary things to establish residency. Bob asked a friend, Josh, what bank would be the best to do business with. Josh had told him that the First National Bank of La Crosse was pretty good. Bob parked in the parking ramp, and we walked from there. The ramp was dark and empty, so I thought it was spooky, especially if I was alone. I only parked there once when I was alone. But with Bob, I felt safe, and we walked through it arm in arm until we got to the stairs, where he opened the door for me, and I went down first. From there, we walked out onto the street to Main Street where the bank was supposed to be. Bob asked me if it was the First Bank that Josh had said. I told him I didn't remember, but that sounded good to me. So, we walked to the bank to start a checking account. Although it was cold, the wind was not blowing, and I tolerated it better. When we walked into the bank, Bob told the teller why we were there. She said she had to have another person handle it so asked us to wait. We sat down on the plush royal blue chairs, but I got restless waiting and went to the show window where they had everything from cameras to microwave ovens. I glanced at all the things and then returned and sat next to Bob.

Shortly after, a woman came, introduced herself, and said, "Welcome, you'd like to start an account here?"

Bob said, "Yes."

She said, "Follow me." She took us to a large desk where the two of us could sit comfortably and talk to her. She gave us some forms to fill out and told us that she had some unfinished business upstairs to attend to while we filled out the form. When she came back, she explained everything to us including FastBank. When she finished her explanation, she asked us if we would like a FastBank card. We said that we would and said that we would have to pick four numbers for a code number. Bob told me to choose. I said, "What about the last four numbers of my social security number? That would be easy to remember." But I didn't remember and told her 5992 instead of 2992.

She also told us that if we entered a certain amount of money in our account, we could have one of the prizes in the window. The more you put in, the more you can get. Then, she took us to the FastBank machine to show us how to use it, making a deposit on our account.

"But if you forget," she said, "there are instructions and buttons that light up and tell you what to do." Next, she took us to the show window to choose the gift we wanted. I had no hesitation in deciding which one I wanted. I had always liked and wanted a bentwood rocker. It was a little more than the credit given us, but for a small price we could have it, and Bob didn't mind. It was too big to put into the Pinto, so we told the lady that I would come back for it next week.

We headed to Viroqua to pick up the children and had lunch there. We left early, so we could start unpacking and sorting out what we needed and what could be stored. The problem was that some of the boxes were unmarked. But it was kind of fun, kind of like Christmas, with many surprises.

The trips back and forth from La Crosse to Viroqua were not pleasant for me. The kids would fight or yell in the car, which would precipitate or intensify a headache. Then, I'd be irritable with them. Sometimes, I would try to meditate the headache away instead of yelling at them. But it was very hard to meditate in a noisy car. So usually, my headache was still there when we got to our destination. I did not however give up on the meditation; I wanted to get rid of the tumor as well as relieve the headache.

CHAPTER 9

During our first few weeks in Wisconsin, I became preoccupied with thoughts about the remaining tumor. It became an obsession. I talked to Bob incessantly about it. I knew I had to contact Dr. Anderson in La Crosse, but I was dreading it. The trips from Viroqua to La Crosse and back worried me. I experienced strange sensations in my head which I believed to be due to the tumor, but which was probably due to the changes of pressure in my ears when going up and down those coulees, but which was not relieved by yawning with my mouth open. I decided to meditate in order to cope with these feelings, which felt much like a roller coaster in my head. It was not a fast feeling, but it did have up and down sensations. Although it was not easy, I kept trying to imagine those sharks eating the tumor. It was particularly hard when I had a headache.

During the first three days that we stayed with my in-laws, I had asked Bob if I should give Gundersen a call. He told me to give it time; that my records probably hadn't reached them yet. I was relieved, yet ambivalent about his answer. I wanted six weeks in which to meditate and cure my tumor. I believed that it would take six weeks because a patient in the book had done it in six weeks. On the other hand, I was leery of waiting too long. Dr. Golden had said he'd call Dr. Anderson and tell him that I was coming. The first week we also had to put in a phone. Actually, there was already one in the apartment, but we had to have the service put in our name.

Ken had been very restless and quite belligerent, especially since I had arrived. Moving to the apartment was a little [better], but not much better, since it was still crowded compared to our fifteen hundred-square-foot home in Albuquerque. Ken was very wild and active, and I was anxious to get him back into school. It was still hard for me to deal with such activity. I still believed that a Catholic school would be best for him since they provided somewhat more discipline. So, Bob and I looked through the phone book, and Bob, knowing La Crosse better than I, said that St. Pius X sounded the closest. So, the next week, I called the school and made an appointment to register him.

I was told that I'd have to meet with the pastor of the parish and register. The parishioners were allowed to "donate" a lower tuition rate. The nun who was assisting the priest said that the suggested tuition was actually put in the Sunday offering. Finding St. Pius X School was not hard. It was not far from Sherwood Manor.[29] One of the back roads actually led to the school, but I didn't know that until I started riding my bike through there. So, I went up Mormon Coulee Road, turned left at the first stoplight, and then went all the way up the little road to the school. I took the kids with me. Ken and Karen had fun going up and down the steps.

The Sister had told us to meet her in the office just right of the stairs. She asked some questions about Ken and then handed me some forms to fill out. While I was filling out the forms, she said she'd call in the pastor to talk with us. She asked Ken if he'd like to go to his classroom to meet his teacher and see his new classroom. Ken, being a little shy and not so eager to start school so soon, rejected the offer. She said that it was okay, that he could meet them all the next day. She also gave me a list of what Ken would need for the rest of the year. Then, she left to get the pastor.

We were seated in a rather large office, in front of a large desk, with the crucifix upon the wall behind the desk, [and] with bookshelves along that wall and on the wall to the right of it. She

---

29 Sherwood Manor is a neighborhood on the South side of La Crosse, WI where Sandra lived when she initially moved to Wisconsin.

came back with an elderly priest and introduced him.

She said, "Mrs. Cowen, this is Monsignor Fitzpatrick."

"Good morning, Mrs. Cowen," he said and extended his hand before I had a chance to correct the sister.

I stood up, shook his hand, and meekly said, "Cowden."

He went behind the desk and looked at the card I had filled out and said, "But, of course." He again looked at the card, after adjusting his wire-rimmed round glasses on his nose. Looking up from the card, he said, "Ah-h from New Mexico. What brings you to Wisconsin?"

"Bob wanted the kids to spend some time with his folks while they are still young."

"They live in La Crosse?"

"No, Viroqua."

He continued asking questions about birth dates and whether the children were baptized. He noticed that we were married in the Newman Center. Then he asked if Bob was Catholic. I answered, "No." He said, "Ah-h, Lutheran." I said, "No, Church of Christ."

Having the information he wanted, he asked Sister to bring in the schedule of fees. A suggested fee was requested, but it was explained to me that we could put it in the Sunday collection in any amount; just so that it was all paid by the end of the year. He asked Sister to prorate it for the time remaining for Ken to be there. She gave me a figure. I told her I could give $20, then put the rest of it in the Sunday collection.

Father then turned to Ken and said, "So you're going to be in first grade?"

Ken wasn't talking much, so I interrupted and said, "No, kindergarten." He had wondered why Ken had gone to school before and wasn't in first grade. I reminded him that he was just completing the last half of his kindergarten year.

"Oh, yes," he said. He welcomed Ken to St. Pius X and let Sister take over from there. She said that Ms. Amber would be his teacher, and then asked me if I would like a tour. I said yes. We walked down the hall, first to Ms. Amber's room, where she called Ms. Amber out of her room for a little while to introduce Ken and me to her, and Karen of course who would not let herself be forgotten. She then showed us the kindergarten lockers, which were more like cubbies than lockers, but she told Ken that next week, one of the lockers would be his and have his name on it. She also took us down to the gym and showed us where they had their physical education once a week.

She then asked where I was living, to see if she could get Ms. Amber to give me some numbers of some other mothers who lived in the area who I could carpool with. I thought that was very nice.

The rest of the week was spent grocery shopping and doing laundry. I called Lovelace to have them mail my disability insurance payments to the apartment.

CHAPTER 10

Three weeks lingered on. Since Bob had suggested waiting on calling the doctor, I procrastinated in calling him because I was now to the point that I was starting to believe that I could cure my tumor and I was beginning to get determined to do it. There was an example of a man in the book who had cured his tumor in six weeks. So, in my mind, I believed that it would take six weeks to dissolve my tumor. So, it was the last week in March that I called Dr. Anderson.

The first three weeks were not without hardships, however. School did not calm Ken down much, especially at home. Every night was a sleepless night until the wee hours of the morning. There was a lot of sibling rivalry and I also had to think of the kids' birthdays, which were coming up.

I'd wake up each morning and meditate. I'd imagine the sharks attacking the tumor. I had remembered seeing Jaws and would imagine that my tumor was the cage in which the man was in, and the shark destroyed both the steel cage and the man. It was sometimes hard to meditate first thing as the kids woke up at about 6:30 and wanted breakfast. Bob was helpful and sometimes would fix them breakfast when he wasn't working and tell them, "Let your mother meditate." I'd try to meditate three times a day for at least fifteen minutes. The most difficult one to do was in the middle of the day. I tried meditating between 10 a.m. and noon. The problem was the noise. Children can make a lot of noise. When

Ken was home, the noise more than doubled.

Ken had to be in school by eight, which meant I had to get up at six thirty and have both kids dressed and fed and ready to go by eight, especially the first week when I drove myself all week. When I got back, and [if] Karen was undemanding, I could meditate peacefully.

Friday evening, March 6th, I got a phone call, which surprised me because I hadn't met anyone in the area yet. She explained that she was Mrs. Hanson, Richie's mother; and that Richie was one of the boys in Ken's kindergarten class. She explained that Ms. Amber had called and told her that I was interested in carpooling, and the other mothers could carpool with me since I lived in the area. She said that she and another mother were carpooling, but that Tony, the other boy, went to the public school, which was not too far. She asked if I was interested in joining them. Of course, I was. She said she could drive Mondays and Tuesdays, the other woman could drive Wednesdays, I could drive Thursdays, and we could alternate Fridays. I told her that was fine with me. I told her I didn't know how to get to the public school. She gave me directions and said it was easy but if I had difficulty, Tony could help me. The school was on the other side of Mormon Coulee Road.

Life in the apartment was hard. Ken was difficult to handle. He and Karen would fight, and I'd send them to their rooms for a "break." Originally it was a "time-out", but Ken had changed the words. He would refuse to go and then threaten to break something or hit me if I threatened to spank him. He mostly got irate when I wanted him to pick up his room which was a total disaster with toys and dirty clothes everywhere. He had gotten the idea that he could do almost anything when I was over-sedated with Tegretol, and he did what he wanted while I slept. The problem was that he'd leave the house without telling me or asking me permission, and naturally, I'd worry and eventually get furious. In Albuquerque, it was not too much of a problem because he was usually at Sally's or Mr. Henson's house. But here I didn't know the people. There were lots of kids, some good and some bad.

The nights were terrifying and endless it seemed. Sometimes, I just couldn't get to sleep and other times I'd wake up shaking from unknown fear. At those times, I'd want to be close, very close, to Bob. And those lines would run through my mind again-"I want to hold you till I die, till we both break down and cry, I want to hold you till the fear in me subsides." But I couldn't hold Bob all night. He needed the sleep. He was working. I needed the sleep too but couldn't seem to get it. So, after getting as near to Bob as I could, I would get up and walk around the apartment and I usually ended up on the couch. I could find comfort from Bob while he was awake, but once he was asleep I just couldn't find it. As uncomfortable as the couch was, I found some comfort in it perhaps because I cradled myself into its corner and I had a false sense of being held. Then sometimes I'd fall asleep in the wee hours of the morning. Sometimes when my anxiety got too high, and I thought I would not sleep all night I would take a valium that I had left over from the hospital. But I was very careful with them, only taking them when I thought it was absolutely necessary. I had read *I'm Dancing as Fast as I Can* and didn't want to follow that path. Occasionally, Bob would have to urge me to take one, because I was so cautious.

In the daytime, it was easier to deal with my anxieties because I was busier. During the week, I would wake Ken at seven for school, give him breakfast, and take him and the other two boys to school if it was my turn to drive. If it wasn't my turn, we would wait for the driver. I would feed Karen if she got up later than Ken. Then, I would go back to bed if I could possibly get away with it as I wasn't getting much sleep. If I did not meditate immediately when I got up, I'd go back to bed, pile the pillows on the wall to support my back, and relax, and meditate. If I wanted more sleep, I'd let Karen in with me.

I didn't start the radiation treatments until the end of April, so the rest of my days in March and April were your everyday mediocre housewife sort of day until Ken came home. Then sometimes all hell would break loose. The most difficult task was getting him to clean his room. When I'd go in to put his clothes away, I'd find wall-to-wall toys and dirty clothes. He didn't want to clean his room, so he'd have a tantrum. He'd run around screaming and yelling at me and sometimes throw things. I didn't know how to handle it, so I'd send him on a "break." It was hard to deal with his hyperactivity and temper when I was under a great deal of stress myself. He was trying to adjust to a new environment. I was trying to survive a brain tumor, a move, and the normal stresses of raising children. I tried to engage his teacher's help in helping me cope at home. But who could believe that such a quiet child at school could be so active at home? Needless to say, our days were hectic but sometimes fun.

Sherwood Manor was located near the La Crosse River and the turtles would crawl out into the street. Sometimes driving was an obstacle course to avoid hitting them. One day Ken came home with one of the turtles. These were not tiny painted turtles. They were about eight inches in diameter and ugly. He wanted it for a pet. I didn't have the heart to tell him no. He only got to see Wilbur, our St. Bernard on weekends that we went to Viroqua. So, I told him that he could keep it for a day and then he could ask his dad whether or not he could have it for a pet. I knew that in the apartment we had no feasible place to keep a turtle of that size alive for long but thought that Bob could convey the message better.

When Bob came home, I informed him that I had allowed Ken to keep it for a day. Ken began begging to keep it. Bob went into a long, sophisticated oration on how the turtle could not survive in the indoor environment and how it would be kinder to let it go back to its natural habitat. Ken was disappointed but agreed to let it go the next day.

The next day, he half-heartedly asked if he could keep it.

"Now," I answered, "You promised your dad you would let it go." With a forlorn look, he left the apartment slowly. His expression was one of grief.

It was not easy for me to make friends in the community as I was so preoccupied with resolving my tumor. The doorbell rang one early afternoon, and I was surprised to have a lady from the Welcome Wagon show up. The Welcome Wagon gave me some free samples of detergent and other household items. She also gave me a cake mix and tickets to a La Crosse play, which we never used. They invited me to a luncheon for new residents at a local hotel. I decided to go. I knew it wasn't healthy to stay home all the time, since I wasn't working. It was on a Saturday, so I left the kids with Bob. I was looking forward to the affair, but it didn't turn out to be that thrilling. Although not old, most of the ladies were older than me and were into dieting, which I wasn't. So, what they had for snacks was made of low-calorie natural and organically grown ingredients. I tasted them but they were not my cup of tea. The brownies were made with soy flour and sunflower seeds. God knows what they used for chocolate! The culmination of the affair was a health film about the four food groups and also about how many calories are in some of our foods such as milk and other dairy products and one piece of steak. Whole wheat bread was advocated heartily but I had been using it for many years. Needless to say, the meeting was disappointingly monotonous to me as a nurse with some nutritional background who didn't need to lose weight.

There was another club in town devoted to the purpose of welcoming new residents. It was called the Newcomer's Club. One of the pharmacist's wives was also a new resident and was going to a social for the Newcomers at the south side of town. Jane called me and offered me a ride to the sponsor's house. She said she would pick me up Sunday night at about 7 p.m.

She rang the doorbell close to seven. Kenny as usual ran to answer the door. He yelled, "Mommy, a lady's here to see you." I told him I knew, put on my jacket, told the family bye, and left. We introduced ourselves and told each other a little about ourselves. I told her I was a nurse and that we had moved from Albuquerque, New Mexico to Wisconsin because Bob wanted his folks to spend some time with the kids while they were still young. She told me she had moved from Illinois, so the weather was not too much different. I thought it was cold.

We arrived at the lady's house at about 7:15. There were two other women there. She introduced me to the two women. There were little candy dishes with mints on the coffee table in front of the green-patterned sofa on which we were seated. The hostess told us to help ourselves and asked us if we wanted coffee. Jane took coffee. I told her I didn't drink coffee, so she offered me a glass of 7-Up, which I accepted. We talked a little while the others arrived. When everyone was there that was expected except one that didn't come, the hostess had each of us introduce ourselves and tell a little about ourselves. When my turn came, I said, "I'm Sandy Cowden. I just moved from Albuquerque, New Mexico and I am a nurse where I worked in OB and Peds." The group was more homogenous. There was another nurse there. They had children approximately the same ages as mine. One lady was pregnant. I felt comfortable talking with them as I felt cognizant about discussing maternal-child topics. I even dispelled some old wives' tales. The meeting ended with a discussion about going out to eat in a French restaurant. The Whiteways Inn, I believe it was called. It was supposed to be fairly expensive, so I bowed out graciously on that one because moving had been expensive, and I hadn't received my first disability insurance check yet. The hostess was most accommodating and gave me her phone number should I change my mind. Unfortunately, I never saw those people again because I didn't attend the dinner and in the following weeks, I was preoccupied with resolving my tumor.

I was desperate to get into a Jazzercise class because the book I was reading said it was most important to be active. So, I started dancing in the apartment some. The book said that the most successful patients were those who ran or actively participated in sports and enjoyed them. I'm not much of an athlete but love dancing so I thought I'd enjoy Jazzercise. I got turned on to Jazzercise when a nurse I worked with said she had to go to her Jazzercise class after selling me a Christmas ornament. At the time I was interested because I had gained two pounds in the hospital and my clothes were starting to get tight. I didn't know how to get into a Jazzercise class in La Crosse, so I took out the phone book and called the YMCA and the Chamber of Commerce. The YMCA told me that they'd send me a newsletter listing the classes, times, and prices. The Chamber of Commerce said they would send me a list of Jazzercise times and places and the leaders' names and phone numbers.

In the meantime, Karen Devine from the real estate company called. She had found out that we were in the area and would eventually be interested in buying a house. Bob told her that we could not buy until we sold our house in Albuquerque. She said that she realized that but wanted to leave her name so that we would consider her when we did want to buy. She also asked if she could be of service in some other way. Bob told her I was looking for a Jazzercise class and asked if she knew of one. She said she didn't but would find out and call me back.

She called back about a week later giving me the names and numbers of the leaders of two Jazzercise classes. I had already received the propaganda of the other places. But I sure thought it was sweet and congenial of her to go out of her way to do something for someone when she knew me only slightly.

I started my Jazzercise in the last week of March. The bulletin had about three classes in the La Crosse area. With Bob's help, I chose the one at the Concordia Dance Hall. One was in Onalaska and the other was close to Minnesota so Bob said the one at Concordia would be the closest. The class was Mondays and Wednesdays at 5 p.m. Bob was usually home by five. If he wasn't, Jack was willing to come over and sit for the kids for an hour. I was only Jazzercising twice a week, so I hinted to Bob that maybe I should have a bicycle so that I could exercise three times a week. He said we didn't have the money. I was sort of disappointed but understood.

The fourth week of March I called Dr. Anderson. I procrastinated making an appointment to see him as long as I thought possible. I believe it would take six weeks to dissolve my tumor and I wanted the best possible chance of accomplishing it. When I called Dr. Anderson, he said he had heard from Dr. Golden that I was the one who had a Grade 3 brain tumor. I told him that my doctors had told me I had a Grade 2 tumor. He insisted he had been informed it was Grade 3.

An awesome fear descended upon me for fear the doctors in Albuquerque had shielded me from hearing the grave news. I was on the edge all day until Bob came home. When he got home, I told him about my conversation with Dr. Anderson. I asked him if he thought of Drs. Golden and Smith were just saying it was Grade 3 to "cover their asses."

He said, "Probably, they're not supposed to accept anyone with less than a Grade 3 tumor.

"But what if we've been deceived and there is a Grade 2 tumor after all," I inquired. "Wouldn't it be wise to buy the bike so I can exercise three times a week just in case?"

One day Bob surprised me with a ten-speed bicycle. I was thrilled and relieved. My hope was renewed, and I started to believe I could beat the tumor. But I needed the help of *Getting Well Again*. I was determined to try. I read and reread the man's testimony of how he cured himself. The first few weeks of riding were cold and uncomfortable, but I'd don my gloves, down jacket, scarf, and cap and set out to ride. The first ride, it was not the cold that was so uncomfortable, but the fact that I hadn't yet built the stamina to ride a great distance without tiring easily. I heeded Bob's warning and did not try to ride a mile the first day. I started out for about an hour, but after eight or nine minutes of riding, I would have to stop and rest. The second week I increased my riding time to fifteen minutes before I'd have to rest. When I went out for my bike rides, I would imagine the sharks eating my tumor again. The book mentioned that the reason exercise was so important in dissolving tumors was that studies had shown that vigorous exercise caused a lymphocytosis on increased production of lymphocytes in the blood. (Lymphocytes are white blood cells that destroy foreign material in your body). So, I also imagined that I was producing hundreds of thousands of lymphocytes.

My initiation to Wisconsin wasn't all bad. I called my friend Sue. We had worked together in pediatrics in Albuquerque for eight years. But we always kept in touch at Christmas and whenever I was in Wisconsin, or she was in Albuquerque. Sue and Dick lived in Brownsville, MN, only about five miles from La Crosse. When we moved to our apartment, I asked her if she could come down on a Saturday so we could go shopping and she could orient me to La Crosse. I gave her directions on how to get to the apartment and she did well until she went right past our apartment. I had told her it was 2501 Scarlett Dr. and she only saw the 2500 numbering on the door and went past to find 2501. When there was no 2501 down the road, and since our apartment was the last one on the block, she returned. I was glad to see her. A familiar face was a ray of sunshine in my time of need.

Sue's mother amused me. The middle-aged spunky woman went through the ½ price shoe sale with all the enthusiasm of a teenager. The shoes were piled in a heap on a low platform table, with no semblance of order. But Mrs. White knew what she wanted and sorted through quickly and efficiently. I also admired her sense of humor. She picked out two pairs of shoes, paid for them, and then we left. We went on to the household department where Sue found some placemats she liked on sale.

From downtown La Crosse we went to Valley View Mall. I don't remember buying anything. The sheer diversion from family life and my absorption with myself was worth the trip for me. I enjoyed listening to Sue and her mother share anecdotes about themselves and the rest of their family. Sue has eight siblings. Although I told Sue what had happened, we didn't focus on that, and our trip was a breath of fresh air in my present stale existence. She did share her own frightening crisis with me. One night she felt a palpitation in her heart. Her husband didn't take her seriously thinking she was making it up. She finally convinced him to take her to the hospital where they ran an EKG strip. She had been experiencing some PVCs (premature ventricular contractions-abnormal heartbeats) and they wanted her to spend the night in the CCU (cardiac care unit), but she refused. Fortunately, it must have been caused by some stress, which once relieved disappeared.

Sue asked me about Mexican food. She didn't care much for the food at Esteban's. And what she remembered most was Presbyterian Hospital's version of Mexican food. She also didn't like it too hot. I told her that the food at the hospital wasn't Mexican food. It was artificial Mexican food. Then, I asked her if she had any plans for next Saturday. She said she didn't, so I asked her and Dick to come over that evening and I'd fix a big Mexican dinner with the works.

My dinner on Saturday, March 14th was a success. Bob helped me and we had gourmet Mexican food. We fixed the works: tacos, enchiladas, tortillas which could be used for burritos as well as beans, ground beef and cheese, lettuce, onions, and green chile as toppings. Sue was a little leery of hot Mexican food, but I assured her that there was also bland food, as I had to fix dinner for the kids too.

After we finished up the dishes, we sat in the living room and talked. We had planned on having them overnight. We put sleeping bags on the floor for Karen and Kelly (their daughter), but the kids just played and made a lot of noise. When they finally got tired, Kelly began to cry saying she did not want to sleep there, so they thought it better to leave.

One of my responsibilities during our early weeks in Wisconsin was to find a good babysitter or daycare center. Since I didn't know any of the neighbors except Mrs. Hanson to say hi to, I looked in the phone book. Elm Grove Day Cancer Center was one of the ones listed and happened to be in the basement of the St. Pius X school, so I called and made an appointment to inspect the center and interview the person in charge. I wanted my children to be well cared for, happy, and have some educational experience too. In early March, I went to inspect the daycare center. Everything was satisfactory except the cost. I found it much higher than I had paid in Albuquerque. They also didn't have hourly rates. They charged through contracts. The older grey-haired woman with her grey hair tied in a knot on the top of her head showed me a list of rates starting from one day a week to full time which was eight hours Monday through Friday. Even if you didn't take your child on contracted days you were charged. I didn't like the terms of the organization, so I didn't commit myself telling her I'd call back if I decided on her daycare center.

I went home and looked in the phone book for other daycare centers. As it turns out, six of them were operated by the same people. There was another daycare center in the La Crosse phone book, so I called them. They too provided services under contract. Much to my chagrin, I settled for Elm Grove Daycare Center. I contracted for two and a half days a week since I thought that was all I could afford.

MY MOTHER'S ROOMMATE

On Friday, March 27th, I had an appointment with Dr. Anderson at 10:30. I was of course apprehensive, as I did not know what to expect. Although Bob was working, he told me to meet him at the pharmacy at Lutheran and he would accompany me there. When I got to the pharmacy, Bob introduced me to his co-workers. Then we walked from the hospital side of the building to the clinic where Dr. Anderson's office was located. When we got there, we informed the young lady at the desk that we were there to see Dr. Anderson. She was a tall, dark-haired lady.

She said, "The Cowdens are here." Then, she handed me a form to fill out and some pamphlets on brain tumors. We sat down on dark green vinyl and steel chromed chairs. I filled out the forms and put down my New Mexico Blue Cross/Blue Shield number. We had obtained extra insurance on me before I left so that I would be covered from the time Bob's insurance at Lovelace was canceled until the time his insurance at Lutheran took effect.

We waited a while. Then, the nurse who happened to be the same lady at the desk took me to an exam room, measured me, weighed me, and took my blood pressure. I took a deep breath and tried to relax while she took my blood pressure. I felt it was probably up due to nerves. I wondered what it was but refrained from asking her. The nurse left me sitting on the end of the table with one of those short white gowns that open down the backside. I looked around the room anxiously. A few minutes seemed like an eternity. Doctors' offices have frightened me since I was a child when I was diagnosed as having arthritis. [As a child,] I had sat on a table, the door was open, and within my view was an oxygen tank which, at the time, I thought was an iron lung, and I was sure I had polio and they would put me in one of those things.

Dr. Anderson came in a few minutes later and examined me. He listened to my heart and lungs, then proceeded to do the expected repetitious neurological exams. He ran through the same questions.

"Do you have seizure activity now?"

"No, the only seizure I had was the one before the surgery."

As he checked my eyes he asked if I saw double. I answered in the negative. He told me to close my eyes and stand on one foot and then the other. He asked me to close my eyes and touch my nose with first one hand, then the other and to bring my index finger together with my eyes closed. Then he asked me to squeeze his hands and I gave them a good hand squeeze. He backed off; maybe I hurt him a little and said I certainly didn't have any neurological deficit. All the time that I was performing these simple exercises, I was thinking that I ought to do one of my Jazzercise routines right there in his office. That ought to convince him, I thought, that I had more coordination than he did.

Dr. Anderson was a big, obese doctor who could scare an elephant and who, although [he] must have been in his fifties, had the face of a young boy from the 50s with his crew cut coming from that era. But I didn't let him scare me. I had Bob with me and had become more outspoken since my surgery.

I got dressed, and Bob came back to the exam room so he could talk to both of us. When Dr. Anderson came in, he began pacing, still reminding me of a schoolboy who hadn't quite studied enough for his exam. He said that he hadn't received the records yet but that he was told it was a Grade 3 tumor and would recommend radiation, but that he wanted the records before I started. I told him we had been told it was a Grade 2 tumor and that I wanted a CAT scan before any radiation.

He said, "To see if the tumor's still there??" I nodded my head yes. He then said it would be nice if it was gone, but he did not see many that were. At this time in my meditation, I was imagining that the tumor was gone and that I was overjoyed about it, jumping up and down [and] hugging Bob and him. I also imagined Dr. Anderson as being pleased and amazed over the whole thing as if it were a miracle.

He dismissed us on the note that, without the records, he really couldn't tell us much. He would contact us when he got my records. I informed him that I had released my records to Gundersen Clinic and had instructed them to send them here. He said, "Well that's the way it usually goes. We get the records long after they were supposed to be sent."

About two weeks later, Dr. Anderson's secretary called and told me I had an appointment for 9 on March 30th. Then she said, "That's all right isn't it?" It was but there was something disconcerting about being told without being asked if it was convenient first. But on March 30th, Bob and I were there to talk to Dr. Anderson. This time there was no exam. The nurse took us into a large conference room where Dr. Anderson was seated at the head of the table with my files in front of him. She seated Bob and me at his right. She sat on the other side and took notes. It was a formal conference room filled with bookshelves and books on one side and degrees on the other.

"I'm going to let you see all the records because…" he turned three shades of pink… "Well, I once had this difficult patient and I just thought it would be better to lay it all out on the table." I knew who that difficult patient was but once you're a nurse you ask lots of questions and don't sign an informed consent for anything.

Bob and I saw the records and from the records, I could not retrieve any conclusive evidence that my tumor was Grade 2 or Grade 3. The only reference to malignancy was that there were some cells that were aplastic. I expressed my concern to Dr. Anderson about this and the fact that Dr. Smith had informed both Bob and me that it was only Grade 2 and that he recommended radiation therapy only as a preventative measure or insurance.

Dr. Anderson insisted that the tumor was Grade 3 and even if it was Grade 1 or 2 he highly recommended radiation therapy. "Well, if it was Grade 3 and not Grade 2, why would he have told Bob and me that it was Grade 2?"

"I tell my patients the way it is even if it's cruel, no surprises. But some doctors have trouble telling their patients the whole truth, well…maybe because he liked you."

"No, no, he didn't like me." I said, "He treated me like a child and anyone who treats an adult like a child doesn't really like them," I thought but thought I'd better not say that.

"How do I know you're not saying this because…(I couldn't think of the right words, but he finished the sentence for me)."

"That I'm saying this just to protect myself," he grinned as he shook his head.

"Well, I think you are. It only makes sense that you'd want to be sure rather than take a chance and, besides, you don't want to get sued for malpractice."

"I really wish you'd take it. If you want more information on astrocytomas and radiation, why don't you go to the medical library and research it a little for yourself, so you can make an intelligent decision."

"Can I really? How do I get in? Don't I need some sort of identification card or something?"

"Just walk in. It's on the second floor, turn left as you get off the elevator and follow the signs. And if they ask any questions, tell them I sent you."

I again requested a CAT scan and he agreed to have one scheduled for me. I informed him of my iodine allergy. He said he'd have his secretary call me with the time and date, but I was to meet him at his office so I could be premedicated for the probable allergic reaction. He gave me a prescription for some Decadron, which Bob took and filled.

At this point, I had only agreed to the CAT scan and would consider radiation therapy. He also wanted me to meet Dr. Doubont (radiation oncology), but he said that could be done at a later date because I was already going through quite a lot already.

His secretary called me that week and again informed me of my appointment. It was Friday of the same week. They were in a hurry to get me to take the radiation as soon as possible if my life depended on it.

On the appointed day, Bob and I showed up again at Dr. Anderson's office. Dr. Anderson was very concerned about my possible allergic reaction to the contrasting dye, unlike Dr. Smith. I followed his instructions on taking the Decadron the previous night and the next morning.

When we arrived at the office, he had me sit on a stretcher and had his nurse give me an injection of Decadron and Benadryl. He told the scanner technician not to start without him. He was prepared for an anaphylactic reaction. As the medications took effect, I became drowsy and decided to lie down on the stretcher.

I was getting quite sleepy when a girl came to take the stretcher to the basement where the scanner was located. In my dreamy state, I heard Dr. Anderson tell her to tell them not to start until he got there.

I was taken down to the basement and asked to move onto the hard steel table. The technician had the IV ready but did not start it as instructed. I lay on the table for about five minutes nervously anticipating the venipuncture when I remembered this time could be put to good use. I closed my eyes, relaxed, and meditated. I went through the whole scene in my mind: the technician starting the IV, the pictures being taken, holding my head still, and the final result of there being no remaining tumor. In my mind, I was kissing and hugging everyone with joyous relief.

Dr. Anderson came in about fifteen minutes later. He told the girl to go ahead and get it started. She was friendly and asked me if I liked to ski. I told her I'd like to learn but had never had the opportunity, being from New Mexico where the snow accumulation for skiing was a fairly expensive proposition. She said she had some cross-country skis that she wanted to sell. "Well, we're just renting in La Crosse," I said, "but I'll keep you in mind when we get our own place."

She finished taping the IV in places and said she'd be behind the window where I could see her and to wave if I needed anything. I couldn't think of what I could possibly need but I said okay.

Dr. Anderson waited until a few minutes of the solution had gone in and was satisfied that I probably wouldn't have a reaction. The big machine came over my head, clicked, and moved back. The girl came to adjust my head between the two brackets and asked me how I was doing. I said fine except I had an itch on my back I wanted to scratch. She had me sit up and said there was one little welt probably from the IV solution but that they were almost done. So, I laid back while they finished taking pictures.

After a few minutes, I noticed that the IV solution had run out. I waved at the window and the girl came back and asked me what was wrong. I informed her that the bottle was empty. She said it was okay. They were done, and she'd remove it in a minute. Dr. Anderson came in, and she went into the glass room. She showed him the pictures and he seemed happy and excited and said I'd done very well and said he'd talk to Bob and me upstairs in a few minutes. I breathed a sigh of relief and thought that the tumor must be gone.

The girl came back into the room and removed the IV and replaced it with a Band-Aid. She said bye and wished me good luck. They asked me to get back on the stretcher and wheeled me upstairs where Bob was waiting for me. He asked me how it had gone. "Okay, I guess," I replied.

The nurse helped me off the stretcher and told me that, when I got dressed, she would take us to talk to Dr. Anderson. After I got dressed, she led me to a different exam room around the corner. She seated Bob and me on the chairs there and said Dr. Anderson would be with us in a few minutes.

We whispered a little. Bob said, "Nervous?"

I said, "Yeah, a little." He held my hand comforting me. We waited wondering what the news would be. In a few minutes, Dr. Anderson returned with two of the CT scan slides. He placed one on the film viewer and turned on the light and said, "I've decided to show you everything so you can make an informed decision." He also mumbled something about his "difficult" patient.

The convoluted outline of my brain and all the crevices of my brain appeared when he turned on the light on the film viewer. The film was mostly grey with little dots of even coloring. The only darker area was in the middle where the lateral ventricles are located.

He pointed that out to us then said, "The tumor is here." When he entered the room he seemed delighted with the results. He said I'd done great, and I began wondering whether it was the fact that I didn't have a reaction or the results of the film. When he began to show us the film, he pointed out the lateral ventricles and then said the tumor is here moving his finger back and forth over an indistinct area over the midline where he knew the tumor would be. He also showed us the scar from the surgery. I kept getting closer and closer to the viewer as I saw nothing until I almost had my nose on it. I didn't want to call him a liar, so I just listened as he strongly recommended therapy again. He again advised me to talk to Dr. Doubont. Again, I told him I wanted more time to think about it. As he finished his speech, he suggested that I stay and rest until the medication wore off. I said I was okay, and Bob agreed so we left. As we left, I asked Bob, "Did you see anything?"

He said, "No, but I didn't want to say anything in case you saw something." Things didn't appear to be on the level as he reassured me, so I decided to take his offer up on going to the medical library to investigate statistics of survival with or without radiation. I planned to compare CAT films with mine.

The next day, I left Karen at the daycare center after Ken had gone to kindergarten. The library was where Dr. Anderson said it was. It was very quiet as no one was around, so I just went ahead and walked in. The card catalog happened to be close to the entrance and that made it convenient for me. I looked under both topics- astrocytomas and CAT scans. As I was writing the number of the books down, a woman approached me and asked if she could help me. I told her I had found what I needed and thanked her for her offer.

I didn't have much trouble finding the books, although one was missing. I took a couple of books off the shelf to a nearby table. I didn't pay much attention to the statistics, as they were all grim. But I looked over dozens of CAT scan pictures of brain tumors. What I saw were very obvious changes in texture and color where the tumors were in the pictures. I decided that my tumor wasn't there anymore.

CHAPTER 11

I got a letter from her sister saying that she thought radiation would be in my best interest. Only it was written in more of a reprimand and I was infuriated. "How in the hell did she know I was considering not having the radiation?" I asked Bob as I expressed my feelings over it.

It was a very troubled part of my life. It seemed as if everyone was trying to control my life. Even my mother seemed to be expressing her reservations over my rejection of radiation because my tumor was gone. I thought aloud often and when I asked Bob for advice, he said, "They're just concerned about you."

"Well, I don't like the way they're going about it."

"What did Katie tell you to do?"

"Katie didn't tell me to do anything. She just said that it was great that we didn't see anything on the CAT scan."

"Well, what would she have told you to do? Wouldn't she want you to go ahead with the radiation?"

"I guess so."

"And doesn't the book say that you should go along with the treatment, even if you have success with the meditations?"

"Yeah," I said dejectedly. I felt that I had done something great, and nobody was recognizing it, except Katie. I thought she was very smart in not giving advice.

"And what happens if you get depressed?"

"I don't think I will anymore."

"Well, what if I die? And how would you feel if you made the wrong decision."

"You told me you were never going to die," I said in a lighter mood, lifting the conversation up about 90 degrees.

I felt better talking about it, but I couldn't see deciding for the radiation on the account of other people. I decided to make a list of positive and negative aspects of the situation. On the positive side, I'd make the relatives happy, I could be fairly sure that a recurrence would not prevail. On the negative side, I'd lose my hair, I might get sick, and there was always the possibility that I'd never have needed it anyway and the most frightening aspect in the long run was that radiation kills brain cells and does not discriminate between normal cells and abnormal cells. That would mean that I could lose things like memory cells, cells that control coordination and hormonal functions. I needed a better reason than medical and family pressure to decide for the radiation because as far as I was concerned the radiation was only a preventative measure. I did not believe I was going to die.

When I heard from Dr. Anderson that my tumor was Grade 3, I became very frightened and bitter. I now thought that Dr. Smith had lied to me. When I got home, I was determined to find out why he had told me 2 when it was 3. I called Lovelace Medical Center hoping to talk to Dr. Golden because I trusted him more, but I told the operator that I'd talk to Dr. Smith or Dr. Golden when my call was returned. I needed the reassurance that the radiation was only "insurance" as Dr. Smith had put it. I was so distracted that I paced around the apartment until he called back.

When Dr. Smith called back he said, "Mrs. Cowden, is there something I can help you with?"

I said, "You told me that my tumor was Grade 2 and that you recommended radiation therapy just for "insurance."

"No, I told you that it was Grade 3. I told you the truth. I always tell my patients the truth. I never lie to my patients, and I am not starting now."

"You're lying now," I thought. At that, I was beginning to get sick. I managed to say, "You did tell me it was for 'insurance only.' I heard you."

"Sometimes patients hear what they want to hear."

"But Bob heard it too." At this point, I was really sick and started to vomit in the trash can that was by the phone.

"He said, "Mrs. Cowden, Mrs. Cowden...Are you there?"

I finally caught my breath to choke out, "I'm vomiting, my Tegretol level is probably still too high."

I guess he didn't understand me and kept saying, "Mrs. Cowden..." By that time, I was so sick that I did the only thing I could do, since I could no longer talk. I hung up on him.

"That ought to show him how I feel about him," I thought later. Later that night, I told Bob what had happened.

"It just makes me sick (literally) that he lied either then or now," I told him

During my last visit to Dr. Anderson, he told me, "The decision is up to you, but I really do hope you go with the radiation. I have something Dr. Doubont asked me to give you to read. Take it home and read but bring it back in a couple weeks as he wants it back. It was a photocopy of some dreadful statistics correlating brain tumors with and without radiation. The number of deaths according to this piece of material of even Stage I astrocytomas was 97%. The results were frightening. But I remember it was just an election year. I remembered the elections and remembered a reporter saying that statistics were like chicken soup. You could get out of it what you wanted.

The days were hectic and the nights endless. After Bob held me for a while, I'd try to sleep meditating as long as I could. I would see thousands of sharks coming and meeting other sharks at the legs, thighs, abdomen, back, all the way up the spinal cord and chest; they would meet the sharks from the arms at the shoulder and neck and proceed to the brain to devour the tumor even though I believed there was no tumor. When Bob could no longer hold me, I could no longer meditate, I'd pace up and down the apartment. I'd wander up and down the apartment but there was nowhere to go. The quiet of the night increased my anxieties. It was so quiet I could feel my heartbeat and I was so anxious I sometimes had palpitations. I'd finally lie down on the couch and imagined the two sides of the couch that touched me were Bob's arms and he was holding me in the wee hours of the morning as I'd drift off. But usually, my whole body would jerk like a seizure, but I was conscious, and the sensation would sometimes jerk me wide awake and there I'd lie again. I'd watch the sunrise and get nervous about being tired all day, so I'd try to get a few minutes of sleep before I'd have to get Ken up. Sometimes it worked but often it didn't.

The days and nights continued to suck, with me quietly mulling over my indecision over radiation and not so quietly expressing my feelings over what happened to me, and also protesting my objection over Ken's constant running and yelling in the apartment. It went on that way until one day when I received a catalog from the Abby Company. The thing that struck my eye as I flipped the pages was a plaque that had a quotation that said, "A mother can replace anyone, but no one can replace a mother." Right then and there I decided I would go ahead with the radiation. I would not risk a recurrence, for the sake of the children.

I called Dr. Anderson and told him that I had decided to go ahead with the radiation. He answered, "Oh good. That way we can get the rest of the tumor that is thought to be there."

"Uh-huh," I thought to myself. "The tumor isn't there, but he didn't want to tell me. He tried to trick me into having the radiation." He said he would have Dr. Doubont call me.

Bob came home about five that evening, so the first thing I told him was that I had called Dr. Anderson to tell him I'd take the radiation and he said, "The tumor that was thought to be there." I was so relieved that I wasn't even angry with him for trying to trick me into taking the radiation.

I had an appointment with Dr. Dubont. This was the appointment I so dreaded. From the statistics he had sent me, I imagined him to be the sort of doctor who hides his aggressive impulses behind his radiation machine. Again, I nervously waited, sitting on the exam table half-clothed and shivering from cold and fear. Fortunately, he did not take too long (even though it seemed long). He did the usual neuro exam that I had grown accustomed to, with the usual questions as to whether my vision was affected and whether I had seizures and/or headaches. I denied them all except headaches. I answered, "Yes, I still have occasional headaches, but I've got kids too."

I decided to give him a chance. I told him I had seen the CAT scan and I saw nothing and that I'd been meditating and exercising and believed the tumor to be gone.

"The tumor's there," he said adamantly, "I've heard stories about meditating and I haven't seen one case where it worked."

"But..." I choked on the lump forming in my throat.

"It's there," he repeated. "I want to inform you about the side effects of the radiation. The obvious one is that you will lose your hair." I interrupted as this was the only side effect I was interested in for the time being.

"How much hair will I lose?"

"Well, we'll have to radiate to the back of your ears."

"I'd probably lose all of mine and it'd never come back?"

"Some, all, or none of it might grow back. Some actually like their hair better because it's thinner."

"Mine's already thin," I said. "Why can't you just radiate to here?" I put my hand about halfway down/mid-scalp.

"What good would that do?"

"I could comb my hair up to the front."

"It wouldn't look good. Besides, no radiologist would do that. You can go to the Mayo Clinic if you want."

I wanted another opinion, but I knew there was no way I could drive to Rochester and back and have a sane life.

He had me crying by this time, but he showed no sympathy at all and went on to list all the side effects he could think of. He wanted me to sign a consent releasing him from all responsibility for these side effects, which included hair loss, burns, and even brain damage.

I had finally had it with him and told him that if he mentioned one more side effect I'd walk right out that door. Informed consent is one thing but rubbing it in was quite unnecessary. He was a bit shocked and said, "But you do know..."

I shook my head yes. He went out to get the consent form but came right back instead.

"Why all the concern over your hair? Wouldn't you rather be alive than have your hair?" As hard-hearted as he was, I just couldn't tell him that I didn't believe my life was in danger, only my hair. So, I said maybe it has to do with my self-image.

"You could wear a wig."

"But it wouldn't be me."

"We all change."

"I will give you the name of a psychiatrist. Maybe she could help you. It's amazing the things they can do. When do you want to start? Today?"

"No, I'd like to wait till Monday." He told me to go to the basement of the clinic at 10 a.m.

I spent the weekend mostly meditating. The thing I needed to meditate on most was on getting the courage up to actually go. We'd go to Viroqua sometimes on the weekends. At this point in my illness, I felt numb, just going through the motions of daily living and the verge of panic at night. But I knew I had to get through this ordeal, so I would meditate on our little trips up and down the little valleys. Sometimes, I would get a hollow feeling in my head, and this frightened me too. Sometimes, I wondered whether the tumor was still there, despite what Dr. Anderson said and what we saw on the CAT film. The feelings in my head, I learned later, were not due to any tumor, but just pressure changes from the sudden change in altitude exaggerated in my mind.

That weekend I went on meditating, creating in my mind a big machine, as I knew it would be that would attack a tiny piece of "hamburger" destroying it. (The book suggested to imagine the cancer cells as something weak.) I was also frightened by the fact that if the tumor wasn't there, the radiation would damage or kill normal cells.

I didn't know where I was going to leave Karen while I went for treatments, so I called Richie's mother (one of the mothers who car-pooled with me to take the boys to school). She gave me the number of a lady who lived about a block away. I called her and she said she would take her even though she had quite a few children to care for already. I told her I didn't have much choice as I didn't know anyone in La Crosse yet.

One female technician had told me to come at 10:30 because the first session was the longest because they had to measure and mark my head. Monday morning started routinely. I would wake up to the alarm. I'd fluff up the pillows between me and the headboard to get into a comfortable position for meditating. I had stopped meditating on how happy everyone would be when they found no tumor, including Bob and the doctors. I had imagined my jumping up and down with excitement and Bob hugging me while the doctors looked down. Now, I had to change my imagery to gain the courage to take the treatments and [I was] imagining that the x-rays were attaching to the tumor. But I still imagined Bob and I being happy about my "muscle."

After meditating, I got breakfast for the kids and sent Ken off with his carpool. At 9:30 I drove around the block to the address of the lady's house. I started out a little early as I hadn't met her and neither had Karen and I did not know how she would react to a new babysitter. I looked at the address and stopped in front of a small, green house. We got out of the car and walked up the sidewalk. I rang the doorbell and a small lady with brown hair answered. The door opened into a living room, and the TV was on the left-hand side of the room. There were about five children in the room. One was a baby, and one was a toddler crying. Karen was apprehensive since she liked babies. I tried to get her interested in the baby so she could forget her fear of my leaving her.

She still didn't want to stay, but she wasn't crying so I kissed and hugged her and reassured her that I'd be back soon. I bid her goodbye and left the mournful little girl.

But my mind quickly drifted back to my own apprehension over receiving the radiation. I walked down the sidewalk to the car.

Epilogue
By Dr. Karen Cowden Dahl

This was my mother's last written contribution to her memoir. Her words were poignant since the last thoughts that she put down on paper were her saying goodbye to me. She never finished her manuscript. Writing about her experiences gave my mom the strength and confidence to deal with her trauma. Writing was cathartic. She intended to help other cancer patients by sharing her experiences. Ultimately, I hope that I am my mother's legacy, and I will pass on her pain, wisdom, and courage via her words.

My mother's writings ended soon after we moved to La Crosse in 1981. She went on to live over four more years, continuing radiation in Wisconsin. After about six months, we moved out of the apartment in La Crosse. We moved to a nearby town, Bangor, where we had a house on almost two acres of land. My mom continued her nursing career at the Veterans Affairs hospital in Tomah, WI. My brother attended school in Bangor. My dad worked nights at a pharmacy in La Crosse while my mom worked days. By working different hours, one of my parents could be home with me during the day.

Wisconsin winters were harsh. Subzero temperatures and several feet of snow were new to us. My brother and I loved playing in the snow. We had fun exploring our giant yard and the woods behind the house. My mom took up cross-country skiing. We settled into a relatively normal life. My mom accomplished many of her goals. In addition to skiing, my mom began to make macramé. She made the macramé swing for Katie's baby. She made macramé baby mobiles for her niece and nephew who were born when we lived in Wisconsin. Years later when I had my son, my aunt gave me the green macramé mobile with ceramic animals that my mom had made for my cousin. It is still one of my most treasured gifts. The mobile hangs in my youngest daughter's room. After a couple of years in Wisconsin, my mom desired to return to New Mexico. We moved back to Albuquerque in the summer of 1983.

At first, we lived in a rental house on Nova Court on the west side of Albuquerque. We did not buy a house right away since our house in Wisconsin took a long time to sell. I began kindergarten in 1983 and my brother started third grade at a nearby public school called Chaparral Elementary. The following year, when I entered first grade and my brother entered fourth grade, we attended Catholic school. San Felipe de Neri in Old Town Albuquerque was the first school in Albuquerque (founded in 1881). It was also the same school that my mom and her siblings attended. It was the same school where my mother was chastised as a kindergartener for not speaking English. As a first grader at San Felipe, I was also finally old enough for Girl Scouts and earning badges.

In June of 1985, we finally bought a house in Northeast Heights (the part of Albuquerque near the mountains). Our house on Esther Avenue even had a pool. My brother and I started at Arroyo del Oso Elementary, another new school. In second grade, I was beginning my third school in three years. My brother started his sixth school as a fifth grader. My new Girl Scouts troop allowed me to make new friends and have time to be out of the house having fun.

Everyone always said my mom was quiet and shy. Yet, that is not a characteristic that I saw. In fact, my mom tried to find me friends. Right after moving to our new house on Esther, my mom noticed a little girl about my age across the street. She marched me over there and introduced me to her and her mom. Shari is still a dear friend today.

Over the summer of 1985, my mom's behavior changed gradually. The Tumor was reemerging. By the start of the school year, Mom was not herself. She became forgetful. One day we went to McDonald's. She couldn't figure out how to get the speaker to be activated in the drive-thru. We had to get out of the car and jump on the cord. Another time, my mother had trouble with the car when we were out and about. She pulled off somewhere to ask someone to help. The parking brake was engaged. When my mom did something out of character, my dad would simply explain that it was not my mom, it was The Tumor. From summer to fall of 1985, I watched The Tumor slowly possess my mom. It took her ability to take care of me. My dad sent me to get my mom for dinner one evening as she was showering. She was sitting on the floor of the shower. I told my mom that it was dinner time. Then she shut the shower door on my head. Only being seven, I was sad and confused. I didn't know why my mom would hurt me. Again, my dad reiterated that it was The Tumor. I knew The Tumor was kidnapping my mom. The Tumor was conducting a slow, painful lobotomy that erased the personality of a loving, courageous woman. All I have left of my mom are short memories. My only remaining window to my mom's personality is the pages you are holding or reading on your screen.

Second grade was a traumatic year. It will always be a triumvirate of evil consisting of a new school, my mom's death, and watching the Challenger explode on live TV two months after my mom's death. However, when I started school in August, I didn't know what the year would bring. I always loved school, and I made friends in class, in Girl Scouts, and in my neighborhood. In my second-grade class, we made get-well cards for a classmate's mom when she had some illness. I insisted to my teacher that my mom get cards too since she was sick. I don't think either of us knew that my mom would be dying soon… I just knew my mom was sick and deserved cards. Just as Girl Scouts taught me, I found a way to comfort my mom. My mom held and cherished the homemade cards from my class even though she couldn't read them well.

The last five months of my mom's life were hard to watch. I cannot imagine the terror and confusion that she experienced. I also imagine that her mind became a prison. Her disease trapped the brave woman that subpoenaed sharks to eat her tumor. As The Tumor enslaved her brain, it also hijacked her body. She lost the ability to eat, talk, and eventually get around well. She could not wear contacts and had a harder time seeing. As the tumor silenced her thoughts, Mom's soul reached out to us with her eyes and touch. The love was still there. Long after her last spoken word, Mom would squeeze my hand. That was how we communicated. "Squeeze my hand one time for yes and two times for no." Mom was there until the end in some form. My mother's roommate, even in the frontal lobes of the brain, could not destroy love.

My mom occasionally had visitors like her sister and her parents, and of course, her best friend, Katie. Though, I don't recall her family visiting too much. In retrospect, I think it was too hard for them to comprehend and accept. In the last weeks and months of my mom's life (I'm not really sure of the timeline), my dad's mother from Wisconsin came to stay with us. Grandma Cowden took care of my mom when she could no longer function independently. Grandma worked in a nursing home and was equipped to take care of my mom in her final days. Ten years later, Grandma Cowden again came to Albuquerque and took care of my mother's mom, Grandma Garcia, when she was dying of cancer. My mom and her mom both died on a Tuesday morning in November (10 years apart) with Grandma Cowden and my dad there for the final breaths.

When my dad knew that the end was near, he sat with me in the yellow comfy chair in our sunken living room and told me that my mom was dying. I simply asked what we would do. His reply was that other family would help us when needed. My dad watched men die in Vietnam. People always say, "War is hell." Cancer patients and families also experience hell. My dad entered yet another Dante-esque ring, one in which he watched the love of his life be slowly dissolved by cancer and then die. At the same time, my dad felt he had no time to grieve as he was rearing two children alone. Dad summoned up the courage he learned in the Navy and protected and loved his kids.

Although this is my mom's story, my dad played such a big role in all that happened to my family. He supported us financially. Dad took care of my mom and looked after my brother and me. After my mom's death, my dad needed a daytime job since he worked nights. He did not want my brother and I alone at night. But we did become latchkey kids, as my dad was often at work before we left for school and worked into the evening. My dad became a single dad. Luckily, Dad was already a good cook and an involved father. I had everything I needed physically, but our home still felt empty. When The Tumor left, it took much of my dad and my brother. Shadows walked our house. Speaking of my mother was not allowed. I did everything I could to please my father. I spent summers at my grandmother's house in Wisconsin. This gave my dad a few months of relief from single parenting. Growing up without a mother, and in a vacuum of affection, was not easy. I was invisible. I invented ways to get noticed but never found a way. After a few years, my dad was on jury duty with a high school classmate of his. The pair eventually dated and married. I am forever grateful that he chatted up an old classmate. My bonus mom has become one of my very best friends. Nearly forty years after my mom died, I can see how much my dad still misses my mom. His eyes tear up and his voice changes when we talk about her. True love is the most beautiful badge one can earn.

Hallucinations or Reality?

Just as Girl Scouts learn new skills to earn badges, I began the quest to learn who my mom was and become her badge of honor. My dad gave me my mom's writings when I became an adult. He knew someday that I would be her conduit to achieve her book, her final badge. I remember little about my mom. Most of what I know came from typing up her words. As I typed, I saw her face and felt her thoughts racing around in my head. I empathized with her frustrations with doctors. I heard their misogynistic and callous voices. I saw doctors avoid eye contact with a female, Hispanic patient as they preferred to address my dad. I internalized my mom's experiences, pain, and hope. Finally, I organized her thoughts as best I could and finalized her final merit badge.

Badges are not easy to earn. One of the hardest parts of this book was trying to decipher reality from confusion. Much of my mom's memories were written after the fact when she was trying to recall traumatic events and time periods. My mom had a seizure, brain surgery, medication overdose, and this was all a result of a frontal lobe glioma (The Tumor). The frontal lobes are responsible for behavior, personality, and voluntary movement. Frontal lobes play a role in memories. Some of my mother's story may not be entirely accurate. Some of Mom's reality was not real. Her writings are composed of redundancies, inconsistencies, and problematic timelines. Many chapters were well-constructed and linear. Other excerpts were hard to place in time.

My mom's feelings were real, but some memories may be impacted by confusion, hallucinations, or side effects of the tumor. Mom struggled with her cancer diagnosis. She initially states she had a Grade 2 tumor, which has a better prognosis. Then, she wrote she had a Grade 2 tumor with a small amount of Grade 3. Later, she insists that it was only Grade 2 and that doctors were lying to her. There is no way to validate any details. However, I am suspicious that my mother did not understand or believe the diagnosis, or her altered mental status impacted her reality or memory. Astrocytoma tumors, even Grade 2, have a very low survival rate with median survival being three to eight years in 2022. It was hard for me to believe that a doctor would say that she would live for decades, or that radiation was "just for insurance." Even forty-two years ago, a neurosurgeon or oncologist would know that her illness was likely terminal. My mom needed to believe that the tumor was not deadly, or that her meditation would cure her tumor. My mom fervently denied she had cancer. She hallucinated hope. We all need hope. My mom was a fighter and wanted to live for her children. Her dedication to surviving in the face of pain and trauma inspires me to this day. She experienced so much fear, but all I see is courage.

I continued in Girl Scouts off and on until high school. I moved several more times and attended different schools. Moving made sticking with activities such as Girl Scouts difficult. However, there are two things that Girl Scouts taught me that are constant pillars in my life. The first is to always help others. The second is to always keep learning and acquiring skills. Since cancer is a major character in my life, it became my nemesis. I decided at fifteen years of age that I would be a scientist and study the causes of cancer and how to cure cancer and/or reduce suffering. My first badge to earn was a college degree. I earned my Bachelor of Science in Cell and Molecular Biology. While in college, I worked in a lab under a Howard Hughes fellowship where I studied colon and skin cancer. I had very little money for college, so I took a heavy course load and finished college in three years while working twenty hours a week in the lab. Immediately following graduation, I began working on the next badge, my Ph.D. I attended graduate school at the University of Pennsylvania and studied cell growth and cancer. My research focus for the past nineteen years has been ovarian cancer. My goals are to help women by understanding how cancer spreads and becomes resistant to therapy. I continue to accumulate badges in the form of papers and grants. Dissemination of knowledge is the best way I can serve God and my country and help others.

Optimism and the Reality of Cancer Today

According to the American Cancer Society, around 18,280 individuals will die from brain or nervous system tumors this year. Specifically, astrocytoma has very poor survival rates. Patients with Grade 2 gliomas have an eight-year median survival; this drops to three to five years with Grade 3, and fifteen months with Grade 4 (glioblastoma). High-grade astrocytomas often recur after treatment/remission, and relapsed tumors are generally higher grade. While these facts are grim, I am encouraged when I think about how far we have come in cancer research since my mom's death in 1985. The five-year survival rate for brain and nervous system cancers increased from 22% between 1975-77 to 33% from 2011-17. For cancer as a whole, the five-year survival rates have increased by 19% since the 1970s. Cancer researchers, oncologists, nurses, and other healthcare professionals are doing something right.

When my mother was diagnosed with cancer a month after turning thirty, no cancer gene had been identified or isolated. We did not know any of the genes that caused or prevented cancer. The first cloning of an oncogene (a cancer-causing gene) was in 1981 in chickens. This gene made a protein kinase (an enzyme we now know drives tumor cells to grow or divide) called "Src". The human Src gene was cloned in 1985, the year my mom died. At the time of my mom's death, there was no specific evidence that linked the human Src with any particular cancer. However, in the last forty years, scientists have generated an amazing understanding of the genetic causes of cancer, types of mutations or genetics associated with individual types of cancer, new treatment options for cancer, and significantly improved cancer therapies. Many types of cancer have incredible survival rates. Since 1975, non-Hodgkin's lymphoma survival has increased by 26%, leukemia by 30%, colon and breast cancer by 15%, and prostate cancer by 30%. Overall, cancer survival has gone from 49% to 69%. (All statistics are from American Cancer Society Facts and Figures 2022.)

We now know specific mutations called translocations that drive leukemia and lymphomas (cancers of the blood). One type of leukemia called chronic myelogenous leukemia (CML) is treated with a daily orange pill that inactivates the kinase (the oncogene) that causes leukemia. Breast cancers are classified according to the expression of several different genes. The expression of these "markers" helps dictate proper treatment. Advancements have been made in every aspect of cancer treatment. Surgeries have become more exact and sophisticated. New types of radiation increase the killing of cancer cells and decrease collateral damage. More effective and less toxic chemotherapies are delivered in a variety of different ways to limit toxicity and increase tumor killing. A variety of targeted therapies are in use. Targeted therapies stop specific activities in tumor cells while having little or less impact on normal tissues in the person's body. Treatments that direct a person's own immune system to attack the tumors are very effective in diseases like lung cancer and the dangerous skin cancer, melanoma. In many cancer patients, we can identify the mutations/DNA changes that drive an individual's cancer progression, then personalized medicine is used to treat the person's cancer. All of these novel treatments are leading to longer survival for patients. It is no illusion that these therapies are working and curing people.

Today, if my mother were in the same situation as she was in 1981, she would have better treatment options and would have lived longer than four years. However, the survival rates for astrocytomas are still poor.[30] The dedication of thousands of scientists over four decades has made the world a better place. Hardworking scientists generated discoveries that spurred clinical trials.[31] Those clinical trials and ones to come are providing cures for cancer and earlier detection.

Much of the progress in cancer research in the last fifty years has been a direct result of the National Cancer Act which was signed by President Nixon in 1971. Nixon's "War on Cancer" improved lives, saved lives, and changed the world for the better. People like me will not stop fighting this war to bring hope for families and treatments to cancer patients. Incredible progress was made in the last fifty-two years. Imagine what the next fifty will bring.

For the past twenty-six years, I conducted cancer research to honor my mom, to serve my country, and to help others. The Tumor is still with me. The Tumor moved in with my family when I was two. Then, The Tumor murdered my mom when I was seven. The Tumor indelibly shaped my childhood, my career, and my passions. I don't know life without cancer. A couple of years after my mom died, cancer took my grandfather, then both of my grandmothers. I did not know that anyone survived cancer as a child. Now, I know of many cancer survivors. My bonus mother, father-in-law, co-workers, students, friends, and many others I have met are proof that cancer can be cured and we can win the War on Cancer.

---

30 Three to eight years median survival for Grades 2-3.
31 Clinical trials are tests or treatments on real patients.

Survivors are the ultimate merit badges for all of the scientists and doctors that work endlessly on cancer research.

The devastation of cancer inspires me to dedicate my life to research. I need something good to come from so much devastation. My research alone will not cure cancer. Cancer is hundreds of different diseases. Each patient is unique. We will need hundreds of cures if not thousands. As a scientist, I work to generate knowledge that will improve cancer treatments and care. Cancer will become a manageable illness, not a death sentence. Cancer care will be individualized. We will help more kids have moms as they grow up. Mitochondria are little engines in our cells that provide energy for our cells, tissue, and organs. We only inherit mitochondria from our mothers. Each mitochondrion in each of my cells is the energy given to me by my mom. My biggest dream in life is not that I cure cancer, it is that I see my kids become adults. They are my success stories. They are my loves. They have the same mitochondria that were in my mom's beating heart. Just as I am my mom's connection to the future, my kids will carry me and their grandmother's legacy.

Every time I see my kids' smiles and hear their voices, I know that love is eternal. ∞

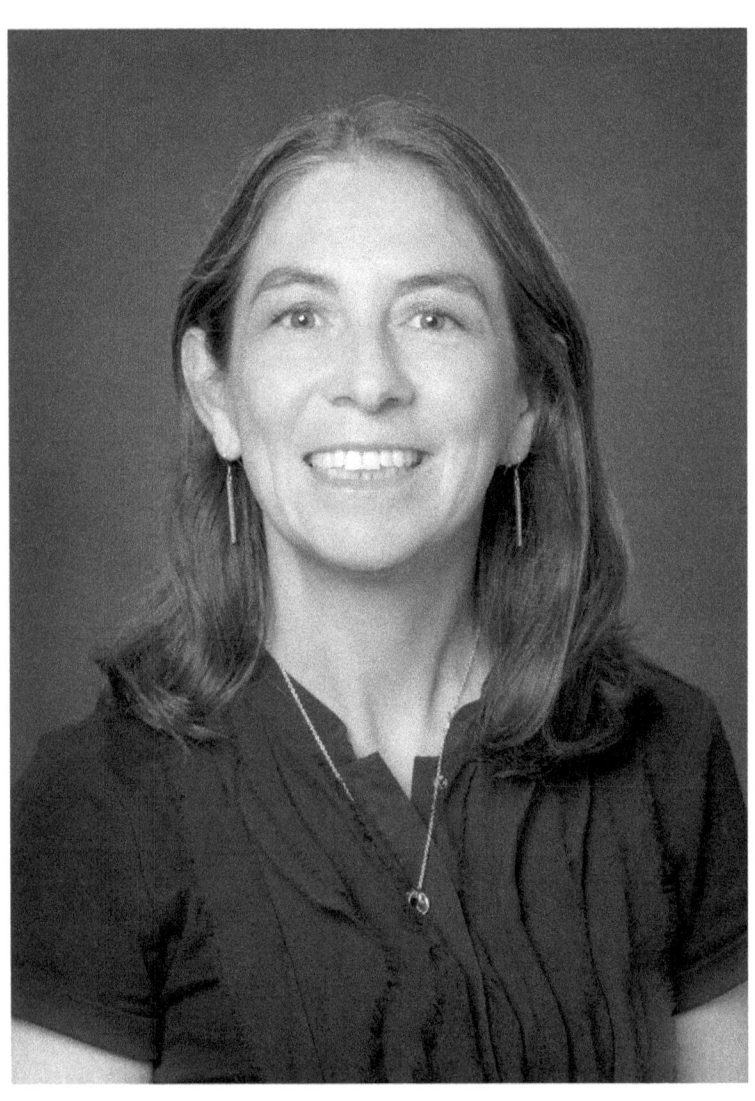

About the Author

Karen Cowden Dahl is a cancer researcher at Gundersen Medical Foundation in La Crosse, Wisconsin with over twenty years of experience in scientific publishing. She earned her Ph.D. in Cell and Molecular Biology at the University of Pennsylvania followed by postdoctoral work at the University of New Mexico. Karen lives in the bluffs near the Mississippi River with her husband and three children. She is an avid runner and can usually be seen at a local race or at her kids' sporting events.

www.ingramcontent.com/pod-product-compliance
Lightning Source LLC
LaVergne TN
LVHW061547070526
838199LV00077B/6932